Yin Deficiency

BURNOUT AND EXHAUSTION - WHAT TO DO!

JONATHAN CLOGSTOUN-WILLMOTT

Frame of Mind Publishing
Edinburgh, Scotland, UK

Contents

Introduction

Unrecognised by modern medicine, Yin deficiency is a disease syndrome recognised in Chinese medicine for thousands of years.

Many modern diseases have it as part of their symptom-picture. It is, unfortunately, a frequent result of living the kind of fast life we live nowadays. However, burning the candle at both ends is not the only way to acquire Yin deficiency. There are a variety of ways, discussed in chapter 4.

Some of the causes of Yin deficiency are hard to guard against. You may even be able to see them approaching and realise that you can do little to prevent them. But for most people options do exist and this book explains them.

Once you understand the concept, commonsense will help you find solutions! This book just points the way. It does show, however, that a huge medical system like Western medicine can overlook a simple idea because it approaches health from a different point of view and is unaware of solutions that were discovered thousands of years ago and have evolved further since then.

This book grew out of my last book, on Qi Stagnation[1], which can certainly worsen symptoms of Yin deficiency. Qi Stagnation, which I had confidently thought would need only 100 pages to cover, in fact took over 500 pages.

1. Qi Stagnation - Signs of Stress, Frame of Mind Publishing 2013. See http://www.acupuncture-points.org/qistagnation.html

So although there was a great deal more that could be said about Yin deficiency, I cut this book down to what was originally a bare 120 pages. I removed an appendix on Social and Political Correlations and shortened other chapters. The intention was to make it short(ish) and easy to read, but above all, **useful**.

However, again to keep the book short, many terms used in Chinese medicine are more fully explained on websites, to which links are provided. The Chinese terms, or syndromes, are a short-hand for conditions of ill-health recognised by Chinese medicine.

There is some repetition so that readers who dip into the book can make sense of passages that would otherwise require going back to earlier chapters. If, like me, you tend to dip into information-type books, this will suit you.

If, on the other hand, you like to read a book through solidly from the first to the last page, I apologise, because you may get a little irritated at reading the same information in several places.

Request!

When you have read this book, may I ask you to review it?

This will help others decide if they might benefit from it. Please post your opinion on Amazon or anywhere else you think would reach prospective readers. Of course I hope you will write a positive or at least a constructive opinion!

However, if you have major reservations or criticisms, do let me know! Then I can improve the book for the next readers. Reach me through my website http://www.acupuncture-points.org, where on many pages there is a way to communicate with me.

Jonathan Clogstoun-Willmott July 2014

CHAPTER 1

What are Yin and Yang?

If you aren't interested in where the idea of Yin and Yang came from, you can skip this chapter and go straight to chapter 2. In any case, this chapter is a bit theoretical, even metaphysical, so if you're not used to it, it can seem a bit heavy.

OK – Still here? Let's get the metaphysics out of the way first before we get down to the practical part!

The idea of a singularity or 'oneness' behind existence is both ancient and modern. Western religions such as Christianity call it God, the Buddhists try not to call it anything, mathematicians say we can never really understand infinity (because you can have as many infinities as you like and you've still got just the one) and astrophysicists just shake their heads because you don't understand.

Unfortunately we lack the mental capacity to understand it. However, we can at least begin to make sense of how it behaves.

Dividing it into Yin and Yang is an ancient way to approach it. Even if you don't yet understand what Yin and Yang are, just let the following sink in or, first, you could read a page on my site about it[1].

---

1. http://www.acupuncture-points.org/yin-and-yang.html

Time and space

These are the Yin places where Yang manifests. In 'The End of Time[2]' the author quotes one of the great early developers of Quantum theory, Paul Dirac, as 'doubting how fundamental the four-dimensional requirement in physics is'.

In other words, time – the fourth dimension – may be unnecessary to explain relativity and quantum physics. In effect, time is an aspect of space and, pushing the boundaries still further, Julian Barbour asserts that it – time – does not exist.

In which case, we only need Space for Yang to manifest.

Yang uses Yin (Time and) Space to manifest. The theory of Change[3] gives Yang the first mover status. Yin exists only because Yang brings it into existence. Space exists because Yang enables it. If you ask many astrophysicists the question 'Before the Big Bang, or the beginning of Time, where was everything?' they will mostly answer either that they don't know, that the question is meaningless or, more precisely, neither 'everything' nor 'space' existed.

My analogy is this: please, just for a few moments, *DO NOT THINK OF A PINK ELEPHANT!*

Now if, inadvertently, you DID think of a pink elephant, how big was it? Was it the size of that Post-It note you keep on your desk? The size of your car? A double-decker bus? The Eiffel Tower? The Moon? Or perhaps it was just against a black background and of indeterminate size. You can make it as big as you like, in fact so big that anyone else looking at it wouldn't be able to recognise it.

And with the aid of your imagination, you can bring it down to the size of a pinhead. It's up to you. Your imagination is versatile

---

2. The End of Time, Julian Barbour, Phoenix, 1999
3. The I Ching, or Book of Change, describes the theory of change. If you like a searching, mathematical explanation of it, read 'Yin-Yang Code' by Ning Lu PhD, pub. www.iuniverse.com. This does, however, challenge the English language in its early chapters. A more traditional but modern translation is 'Yijing, Shamanic Oracle of China' by Richard Bertschinger, pub. Singing Dragon.)

and extremely volatile and you can make the elephant as big as the universe if you like. You decide: your imagination creates only as much space as it needs for your pink elephant.

Your imagination is about the most Yang-like thing you possess.

Life needs a means to live

Just as Yang needs, so creates, Yin space/time to manifest, you need a place to live, to be able to become: your body. (Your Yang not only moves your body but holds it together. After you die, your body decomposes.)

Yin needs Yang to enable life

At the same time, your body needs life (Yang) to enable it to grow, mature and die. Your genes need the life or energy of Yang to evolve over the generations.

Oneness manifests as Yin and Yang

This oneness takes form and life in us. Ancient texts say there is this fundamental 'force' behind existence. Everything is a manifestation as it adapts, twists, turns, and transforms.

Yin and Yang then manifest in us as Qi and Blood

Within the body, there are also subdivisions of Yin and Yang. For convenience Yang is first described as Qi (pronounced *'tchee!'*), Yin as Blood.

Our bodily Qi then takes many subsidiary forms, including Defensive Qi, Inherited Qi, Shen Qi, Stomach Qi, Kidney Qi.

• Defensive Qi is rather like our immune system

- Stomach Qi is the power of the stomach to prepare food for digestion by Spleen Qi
- Kidney Qi is the ability to manage all our inherited and acquired skills and strengths

Blood also takes many forms:

- Repository of personality
- The place where the Kidney function[4] puts into action our inherited and acquired skills and strengths
- Our Reserves etc

As the ancient philosophers developed their thinking, realisation grew that the body had reserves that weren't immediately derived from food eaten and air breathed. They developed the idea of a life essence, inherited from parents and husbanded by the Kidney function. Nowadays in English we describe this as 'Jing-essence[5]'.

Think of it as a small bottle of life energy, received at conception. This is all you get: but you can make a little more of it by living a healthy life. It is precious stuff and you need (they seem to have been vague about some things) 8 pints of Blood to produce one (1) very small drop of Jing-Essence. So increasing your Jing-Essence is difficult.

Using up Jing-Essence is all too easy. Apart from merely using it up as you grow, mature and age, you can accelerate its usage by un-conducive living (drugs; severe illness; shocks; having too much sex – men, or babies close together – women; blood loss; accidents, trauma; lack of sleep; wear and tear etc). All these make your body age faster and in so doing, you use up your supply of Jing-essence.

Ageing means your tissues lose their elasticity and resilience,

4. http://www.acupuncture-points.org/kidney-function.html
5. http://www.acupuncture-points.org/jing-essence.html

your skin dries, you fingernails grow brittle and discoloured, your hair falls, your circulation slows, your brain becomes less resilient and adaptive, your memory goes, your bones break more easily, your hearing reduces and so on. These are signs of reducing Jing-Essence. Jing Essence is about the most Yin thing you've got: your ultimate reserve.

Material properties

In your body, Yin and Yang are 'stored' by Kidney Qi. The body's reserves of Yin and Yang energies, including Jing-Essence are managed by your Kidney function – Kidney Qi.

Kidney Qi, in Chinese medicine, lies behind our capacity for life. In a way, our Kidney Qi manages Yin and Yang in our bodies.

What do Yin and Yang represent in our Bodies?

Yang	Yin
Initiating	Replicating, Multiplying
Moving	Stabilising
Warming	Cooling
Speeding up	Slowing down
Increasing activity	Reducing activity
Dispersing	Consolidating – contracting
De-materialising – destroying	Building material structure
Defending	Nourishing
Back of Body	Front of Body
Upper part of Body	Lower parts of Body
Outside of Body eg skin	Inside Body

When a patient seeks treatment from someone versed in

Chinese medicine, there is a careful assessment of the individual's Yin and Yang energies by consideration of his signs and symptoms – the signs of his dis-ease. These signs can appear on all levels, mental, spiritual, physical, emotional, behavioural, environmental etc.

As a result of disease or ageing, Yin and Yang can each be either in excess or in deficiency.

If Yang is in *excess*, there will probably be too much heat, with restlessness, noise, complaints, fever, tension.

If Yin is *excess*, there will be too many body fluids like phlegm and catarrh, or the body will feel unnaturally cold, slow or heavy, such as during the early stages of a chill.

They can also be Yang *deficiency*[6] which means that we cannot generate enough heat or energy to keep warm, to move, to defend ourselves.

Often in Yang deficiency the upper parts of our body feel more of a burden, cold, heavy and slow.

Yin deficiency is the subject of this book.

6. http://www.acupuncture-points.org/yang-deficiency.html

CHAPTER 2

Yin Deficiency Explained

Lack of nourishing, moistening, supporting, calming, cooling

After exposure to one of the causes described in chapter 4 on Causes of Yin Deficiency, such as a protracted fever, you will feel tired.

Whether you tend, other things being equal, to feel tired and cold, or tired and slightly warm depends on your metabolism – your 'metabolism' being the Western medicine way of explaining it.

In Chinese medicine, which has existed in daily use – and now worldwide – for 3000 years that we are fairly sure about, if when tired you tend to feel cold, you lack Yang: if slightly warm, you lack Yin.

With Yin deficiency it is as if your body's ability to keep itself calm and cool has been damaged.

Keeping cool means both physically and metaphorically. In other words, you may find, with Yin deficiency, that you more easily lose your patience, your 'cool'.

But it goes much further than that. Your body becomes less able to re-nourish itself. Even with good, nourishing food, well-cooked, well-presented, and properly chewed before swallowing, your body may not quickly be able to

- Moisten your skin

- Lubricate your eyes

- Maintain flexibility of mind

- Improve your memory

- Give you the energy you need

- Enable you to rest comfortably and to sleep well

After an exhausting war, such as after either of the two World Wars of the 20th century, the main protagonists, having hurled everything they had at one another, were short of

- People

- Machinery

- Housing

- Money

- Fuel

- Food

- Transport

These are the wherewithal (Yin word) needed to get going again.

People were not short of ideas! Ideas are Yang, and insubstantial, not proved until turned into Yin reality; so, easy to produce.

For example, I can think of any number of ways in which I might be able to make a fortune, but only some kind of application (ie work, a yin-type of process) on my part will bring any of them to reality. In many countries, after those wars, many peoples wanted change from their previous governments. Change at least gives hope (a Yang word).

So to get going, you had to start producing the Yin wherewithal. But before that you had to have an idea (Yang-word) about what to do. Most people just got down to work, re-building their lives. Those with the big Yang ideas became politicians or entrepreneurs.

Where those ideas came to fruition, the government achieved the production of national wealth and the entrepreneurs made money.

Until then, with all the shortages, people died of inclement weather, starvation or poverty. Many people who had endured the privations of war with disease, poor food and overwork took ages to recover. They were less resilient than before. The cupboard was bare.

Not surprisingly, after the first world war, at least, they were more susceptible to disease. Only because of the discovery of antibiotics were we able to reduce the ravages of diseases like tuberculosis after the Second World war.

After any national disaster, resources are poured into repairs or re-building. Ultimately if the replacements are well-considered and not just replacing what was already non-productive, the renewal benefits everyone. New housing is warmer, easier to insulate, less costly than before. New railway lines go where the need is expected to be rather than where they have always gone.

A war is a hugely destructive, creative process (Yang words). It gets rid of masses of old unproductive systems, assets and, dare one say it, of many such people. But replacing them with better 'assets' (Yin-word) takes time.

That time can be years, because Nature takes time to change organically. The farmers of Flanders in Belgium and in the North-East of France, after the first World War, found their fields already ploughed up after the depredations of the war. But before getting to work, a huge effort went into removing the dead, war machinery and munitions. Then energy went into creating farm buildings and habitats. Government money (created by printing money or borrowing or grants from other countries or from savings) was made available, but the work still had to be done, having found the right people to do it.

Once enough people, machinery and seeds were available, fields could be set out, seed planted and Nature given the necessary months needed to grow plants for food. Given (time and) space (yin), the 'life force' (yang) can manifest.

Signs of lack of nourishment, dryness, weakness, warmth

When soil lacks nourishment, plants don't grow. For soil to facilitate growth it needs the raw materials that make good soil, including decaying matter, shit from the worms, ground rock, minerals, and a good fungus undergrowth to extract nutrition and exchange it with sugars from plants. It also needs moisture and warmth, preferably from the sun.

Then it needs a healthy seed, which makes use of these resources.

Any one of these resources, if lacking, stunts growth. Even if the other ingredients are there, the omission of the fungus prevents the seed and its roots from extracting what they need so growth is slower. Any missing ingredient makes the plant more susceptible to disease.

Where the plant is well-nourished and the ground moist, the earth stabilises the plant and its leaves rustle only in the wind.

Without water, any growth is soon stopped, and in time the ground cracks open. If a plant has put down roots into that cracked, parched earth, passing traffic makes the ground shake and the withered leaves tremble.

Similarly, the hands of emaciated old people tend to tremble, unlike those of their healthy, well-fed, grandchildren.

Yin Deficiency easily leads to emaciation, heat, hyper-states

So without the Yin wherewithal, plants are Yin deficient, meaning that they show weak signs such as lack of growth, dryness, poor nourishment, low resilience.

Also, if Yin is deficient, Yang will appear to be in excess, but only because it is not restrained by Yin. So you may get mild yang signs like:

- Trembling or Quivering
- Susceptibility to over-heating or to drying out easily in any warmth
- Haste: growth is unbalanced
- Easily tire or fall
- Hyper growth without resilience
- Emaciation and thinness

As a result such plants don't provide the nutrition that is needed by people eating them. This has become a problem where over-farming has exhausted the soil[1]. In such cases, the soil must be rested and, if necessary, fertilised.

In a world where the resources of earth and sea are being used up faster than they are replaced, farming with artificial fertilisers may be necessary. But those fertilisers have to come from the Earth too, so the better course is to maintain the earth's patency by good husbandry and not making too many demands on it.

The same goes for us, when Yin deficient.

1. http://en.wikipedia.org/wiki/Soil_retrogression_and_degradation

The qualities first mentioned in this chapter of nourishing, moistening, supporting, calming, cooling, are usually associated with the parental function of mothering.

The ancient Chinese don't seem to have been disposed to write big textbooks on the psychological aspects of anything, let alone mothering. However if you know where to look, they did in fact write a good deal about it, but from a different perspective.

This was in comments about the many relationships between Yin and Yang as set out in an ancient Chinese book called I Ching[2], (pronounced Yee Jing). Together with comments about the actions of acupuncture points along some of what are called the Extraordinary channels of acupuncture, and a number of other texts, some Daoist, they did in fact have quite a lot to say.

However, until you become adjusted to how they said it, it's not easy to make sense of. They ascribed much of what we call the mothering function to an acupuncture channel that runs down the mid-line of the front[3] of the thorax and, similarly, the fathering function to the acupuncture channel running down the mid-line of the back[4] of the thorax.

These acupuncture channels are thought to be amongst the very first to be created in the developing foetus. As a result of those early extraordinary channels, (there are in fact eight of them, of which two others are also important early in embryonic development) all the other acupuncture channels eventually come into being.

These two early channels in particular provide a kind of deep resource for all the others. The one down the front, known as Ren Mo (or Ren Mai, depending on where you learn about it)

2. Already alluded to in Chapter 1. There are many translations. Eg I Ching Book of Change, John Blofeld, Unwin 1965
3. Ren Mo, also translated as Directing or Conception channel. http://www.acupuncture-points.org/conception-vessel-points.html
4. Du Mo, also translated as the Governing channel

has many points on it that relate to our nutritional status and capability, and to our personality and personal expression.

If our mother (or whoever supplied that role in our lives) gave us a loving, consistent support from the very earliest stages of life, both within the womb and after birth, we are more likely to have been well-nourished.

That means, in Chinese medicine, that our Blood (capital B to denote what the Chinese mean by the word) would have been dependable, making us personally assured, confident, resourceful, physically strong and resilient, because those qualities go with good Blood.

If that nourishment was lacking, whether in terms of mother's milk, love, attention, succour or encouragement, then our Blood is likely to be less well-structured. We shall then lack in confidence, in resourcefulness, in trustfulness, in personality: we shall easily be discouraged.

When you see someone like this they often don't stand erect or present themselves assuredly. They have personal insecurities. They are more likely to adopt the foetal position in bed, to curl themselves round the front of their thorax protectively, especially when anxious or attacked.

They don't look well-fed, and their eyes lack sparkle. Later in life, they may become aggressive when they haven't learned assertiveness, may search for attention and praise beyond whatever is normal, may become backroom lawyers rather than front-of-house presenters.

Of course, as you will read later, there are other reasons why people become like this, but in terms of where we start from, in the womb and immediately beyond it, the nurturing side of life can either set us on the right path, or not.

These people where the mothering function failed may have a predisposition to Yin deficiency all their lives, or at least until either they have undertaken definite steps in self-development or, because age often brings wisdom and experience, (both Yin-type words), as they become older.

Until then, they may never feel they are properly accepted or acceptable, that their bodies can't supply them with what they need for good, reliable health (hence gastrointestinal problems may dog them for years), and that inner insecurities limit their capability.

Distinguishing between Yin Deficiency and Yang Excess

A vital distinction must be made by anyone treating patients. The ability to distinguish between Yin deficiency and Yang excess can mean the difference between making the patient better or worse.

In Yang excess, there will have been some kind of 'invasion' by something to which your body responds vigorously, usually with inflammation, bruising, heat and/or fever. Although this invasion can come, technically, from an internal source, such as when a bin of compost begins to cook, mostly sources are external, being from bacteria or viruses.

Yin deficiency arises nearly always over time (chapter 4 covers this in much more detail) from protracted disease, working too hard for too long or from exhaustion caused by high fever. Yin deficiency can have signs of fever, but they are very much milder than those of Yang Excess.

With Yang excess the correct treatment is to help the body get rid of the pathogen. With Yin deficiency the correct treatment is to help the body to build itself up and become stronger.

If by mistake a therapist dissipates the body's energy in a case of Yin deficiency because he believes it is actually a case of Yang excess, he may weaken the body still more.

CHAPTER 3

Western Equivalents

Western diseases that often show signs of Yin Deficiency

While the following syndromes 'recognised' in Western medicine share characteristics with Yin deficiency, they are not the same.

Many chronic conditions when they continue indefinitely have features of Yin deficiency. For example, the following often share symptoms with Yin deficiency:

Malnutrition[1]

Poor food, or foods without needed nutritional ingredients, or not enough food, or foods containing substances that either cannot be absorbed or can damage the body, or just poor eating habits, all may lead to malnutrition.

In effect, the body starves.

While humans have often starved or chosen to fast for short periods of time, without danger and often with benefits, prolonged malnutrition means the body cannot repair itself nor function properly. Weight is lost, endurance suffers, immune

1. See http://en.wikipedia.org/wiki/Malnutrition

system weakens and resources are depleted. Organs cease to function properly and eventually you die.

On the way, there are many signs of deficiency, not least of Yin.

Malabsorption syndrome[2] and problems with assimilation of food: like malnutrition, eventually your resources are depleted.

Anaemia[footnote]See   http://en.wikipedia.org/wiki/Anemia[/footnote]: some types.

Auto-immune diseases[3]: the body appears to attack itself. One part cannot defend itself against another.

Metabolic disharmony[4]

Overuse of resources:

- Mental and physical overwork
- Exhausting childbirth
- Excessive sexual activity
- Prolonged fevers
- Weak constitution

Sympathetic/parasympathetic nervous systems[5]

Yin and Yang relate to all aspects of life, so there is also a close relationship with the nervous system. People with Yin deficiency often have an in-efficient parasympathetic nervous system, allowing their sympathetic nervous systems to burn them out.

Sometimes an effect is local or short-lived, such as when a season of very dry, hot weather injures the Lung Yin (see chapter 4). In other cases it has a major, systematic effect. The

2. See http://www.healthline.com/health/malabsorption#Overview1
3. See http://www.nlm.nih.gov/medlineplus/ency/article/000816.htm
4. See http://www.ncbi.nlm.nih.gov/pubmed/11388775
5. See http://en.wikipedia.org/wiki/Nervous_system

latter occurs when, for your particular kind of body and bio-type – your constitution – you have for too long eaten the wrong foods , or taken the wrong amount of exercise (probably too much) or been under too much strain, or put yourself under some other kind of strain that you cannot handle.

Endocrine, especially adrenal insufficiency[6]

People with adrenal insufficiency can show signs of either or both of yin and yang deficiency.

Estrogen deficiency at menopause

As a woman's body changes at the menopause it stops manufacturing Oestrogen often causing hot flashes and mood changes. In some extreme cases, especially where there has been concurrent anxiety or stress, perhaps from relationships or work, these signs of what is called in Chinese medicine 'Empty Heat'[7] lead to destruction of Yin fluids/Blood with symptoms such as skin dryness, reduction in genital fluids and hair loss.

Acid/alkali balance[8]

Acidosis, ie too much acid in the body's fluids, is thought to leech out minerals from bones, making them more brittle and, in effect, less yin. The body often compensates with increased weight. Chronic fatigue – lack of resources – is common. With less of the necessary fluids, digestion is weaker and some unwanted forms of Yin develop such as yeast overgrowth.

---

6. See http://en.wikipedia.org/wiki/Endocrine_disease
7. http://www.acupuncture-points.org/empty-heat-and-cold.html
8. See http://www.betterbones.com/alkalinebalance/ but also http://en.wikipedia.org/wiki/Alkaline_diet

Toxic influences

Modern science has produced fertilisers to encourage more frequent crops than in the past. In so doing it has also produced substances toxic to insects and natural bacteria that normally live on plants. This toxic matter is either absorbed by the plant or runs off onto the earth. If absorbed, we end up eating it, using up our body's (Yin) resources to metabolise it.

Likewise there are many toxic spills by industry into the water supplies and sea, jeopardising the health of future generations. Where exposed to the toxic influences humans are either poisoned or use their resources to detoxify. In either case there is a burden on health resources.

Vitamin/Mineral imbalance

Poor nutrition or poor eating habits contribute to nutritional imbalances. Modern Western diet usually seems to produce excess acidosis in the body, leading to tiredness and burn-out.

Fast/slow oxidisers[9]

Very fast oxidisers can burn out, but it is the slow oxidisers who have reached the exhaustion stage who become more prone to Yin deficiency.

Thyroid/hyperthyroid[10]

After a period of hyperthyroidism, patients typically reach burn out and Yin deficiency.

9. See http://www.drkaslow.com/html/fast_oxidizer_diet.html
10. See http://www.patient.co.uk/health/hyperthyroidism-overactivethyroid

Infectious disease

Yin deficiency can be caused by a series of high or protracted fevers. Yin deficiency does not cause infection but may make it more likely because Yin deficiency often, in time, proceeds to 'Yin deficiency with Empty Heat' in which there is a mild fever and susceptibility to infection.

High Blood Pressure[11]

High Blood Pressure, or Essential hypertension, is often an expression of excess Yang, arising from, say, stress or poor diet and/or lack of exercise. But it can also arise from Yin deficiency. Indeed, both can be involved.

Tachycardia[12]

A fast heartbeat is a sign of increased Yang over Yin. This may be because of circumstances of excess Yang (eg vigorous exercise or excitement) but can also be because of deficient Yin. Or both.

Deterioriation in Body tissues

For example, osteoporosis[13], which occurs when your bones lose vital structural ingredients such as calcium. This tends to occur as you age unless you take enough weight-bearing exercise to encourage your body to maintain healthy bones.

Also, as you age, you create less and lose more muscle, having reached a peak sometime in your twenties. Only by

11. http://www.nhs.uk/Conditions/Blood-pressure-(high)/Pages/Introduction.aspx
12. http://www.medicalnewstoday.com/articles/175241.php
13. See http://www.nhs.uk/Conditions/osteoporosis/Pages/symptoms.aspx

using your muscles physically so that your body is forced to repair them can you begin to reverse this trend.

The above do not exhaust the ways of non-Chinese medicine in which Yin deficiency may be reached!

The next chapter explains the causes of Yin deficiency.

CHAPTER 4

Causes of Yin Deficiency

If you can identify the cause of your Yin deficiency, you will be closer to doing something about it. Having read about the background to this condition in previous chapters, you will realise that others have experienced what you are experiencing. Many of them found ways out of their problems. So probably can you.

The younger you are, the more time you have to recover, and if your health is otherwise good, the faster it will happen.

But although as you age your body's Qi works more slowly, with the right help you can make huge advances in your health even as you get old. However, recovering from Yin deficiency takes both Yin and Yang working together. So husband your Yang energy! Don't do too much, and try not to get physically exhausted.

We can divide the causes of Yin Deficiency into two broad categories (*Internal* and *External*) although, as you will see, the distinction is not always obvious. You will realise that at least one of the causes is plain old-fashioned hard luck.

Either category can drain the yin from the body, an organ,

the Jing essence[1] or the Blood[2], depleting its resilience and eventually reducing it physically so that there is less of it.

INTERNAL CAUSES

Internal causes of Yin deficiency nearly always take time to occur. That means that we often have some control over them.

There is one exception. The exception is 'Full Heat', a febrile condition that can rapidly deplete the body's store of sweat and blood and its ability to regenerate them.

You see it in people of any age, but in young children or babies it can damage them and slow their health maturation down quite a bit. The body throws everything it has into producing a fever to destroy an invading 'bug', and the effort exhausts it.

Constitutional:

Constitutional: Some people are born with constitutions that let them down from the beginning. Sometimes the problem shows itself only later on.

Often one or both parents have had poor health at the time of conception or the mother suffered a difficult pregnancy, perhaps with illness or poor nutrition. But we are much better at keeping people alive than we used to be, assuming the absence of starvation, war and early disaster.

- Premature birth can stop the mother's womb from properly finishing the job, leaving the child with a tendency towards Yin deficiency. This can show as an early tendency to acute episodes of what appear as excess Yang; inflammation and over-reaction to foreign stimuli. Even those born with disadvantaged constitutions can, if they take care and get

1. http://www.acupuncture-points.org/jing-essence.html
2. http://www.acupuncture-points.org/blood.html

help (love, food, support) live with a tendency to Yin deficiency all their lives and remain comparatively disease free into old age, compared with others, blessed with good constitutions who 'blow' it through bad habits.

- The hardest time premature babies have is usually in their teens when their Yang energies, not least in the form of sexual hormones, find themselves unopposed by enough Yin stabilising energies. The teens are hard enough for normal people, let alone those with a constitutional Yin deficiency!

- However, many children not born prematurely also suffer from an excess of Yang energy in their teens. Read more about this in chapter 7 on 'Stages of Life'.

- The mother's health before and during pregnancy is vital for laying the foundations for a secure Yin reserve in life. Stress, worry, major emotional issues, relationship issues, nutritional deficiencies, poisons, electromagnetic influences, diseases: modern science is also waking up to the manifold problems that affect the health of the foetus. But our inherited constitutions are tough. Over 1 million years of evolution have given our genes all sorts of survival strategies. Our problem now may be to allow our genes to continue to evolve, without imposing restrictions on their evolution or trying to maintain a status quo that suits us but may not suit the needs of our descendants.

Shock and trauma

- Frequent sudden disease. Chinese medicine describes this as susceptibility to 'Wind'[3]. Wind can be very destructive. On a hot day, a gentle breeze can be a delight. However, storm force winds and hurricanes have huge power to destroy, and when they act, they act fast. Doors tear off hinges in an

3. See http://www.acupuncture-points.org/wind.html

instant: dustbin lids that have obeyed gravity and kept pests out for years, abruptly become the weapons of malevolent devils, bringing accidents and worse. Trees are snapped off, pylons built to withstand high winds go flying. Similarly, our bodies' reactions to disease pathogens can be sudden and life-threatening. There may not even have to be a discernible pathogen, other than extreme heat, dryness or cold. The body, built to defend itself, does so with acute inflammation. This draws on Yin resources. If prolonged, those assets become seriously depleted.

- Intense disease, especially febrile, as mentioned above, can drain Yin reserves. Older people caught in a hot dry situation may be unable to sweat fast enough to keep cool. They and their bodily fluids become exhausted. Just as someone old can take much longer than someone young to recover from cold or dehydration, the same applies to their experience after intense or prolonged heat.

- Prolonged disease may exhaust Yin. The more intense the body's reaction, the faster the exhaustion, but any disease or condition with even low levels of pain or insomnia may in time exhaust Yin.

- Poisons, if they lead to retching or diarrhoea, prevent the body from absorbing enough nutrients from food. So the body lives on its Yin reserves. If the poison acted more systemically, how it affects Yin reserves depends on circumstances. The more intense the reaction, the faster are Yin reserves reduced.

- Stroke: usually fast-acting and very destructive, like a bad accident. It paralyses one side of the body, preventing Qi[4] from flowing smoothly. Convalescence from a stroke takes time and determination. Physical abilities are reduced, speech and memory affected.

4. See http://www.acupuncture-points.org/qi.html

- Surgery is another kind of shock that produces deficiency, both of Yin and Yang and in particular, often produces Blood Stasis[5], which impedes the flow of Qi, further tiring and exhausting Yin. Tiredness and slowness are common. If there has been blood loss, then until the body has regenerated its supply, any effort requires energy that comes from Yin. The younger you are, the faster you recover. Old people take longer to get over surgery and a big operation can have a devastating effect on their metabolism.

Over-work

- ... including long hours, long travel, especially if frequently across time zones, and if it leads to sleep disturbances. Poor sleep patterns and pressure to work at high intensity are common drains on our Yin resources. Of course, our bodies easily adapt to the occasional travel like this, particularly when on holiday with time to relax. The fitter you are, or the more resilient, the more you can manage.

- Desk-bound and mental effort: this is one of the commonest causes of Yin deficiency. Work isn't bad for us, of course, but long hours without rest, day after day, strains Spleen[6], Qi and Blood[7]. People start getting dizzy on standing up, or have mild black-out episodes as they walk. With lack of exercise comes poor sleep. Blood becomes deficient, followed by Yin.

- Physical over-exertion, especially cardiovascular, for over 45 minutes daily. Physical exertion, such as lifting heavy weights, more commonly depletes Yang, but long periods of cardiovascular effort tend to deplete Yin. You see this in runners whose weight is reduced on purpose to benefit their

5. See http://www.acupuncture-points.org/blood-stasis.html
6. See http://www.acupuncture-points.org/spleen.html
7. See http://www.acupuncture-points.org/blood.html

ability to run distance. But this weight reduction is a form of Yin reduction. If the runners don't take proper rest and sleep, they risk Yin depletion.

- Over-exposure to light. Constant light prevents some people from sleeping properly. Artificial light, as in the 24 –hour day, means people think they need less sleep, or tend to sleep less.

- Over-stimulation for too long, as in keeping awake from drugs or coffee, prevents sleep and time for Blood and Yin recovery. The older you are, the more slowly you recover, which is why war, love, sex and competition favour the young.

Emotions

- Anger, excitement, fear, grief. In themselves, none of these drain Yin, but when they are very intense or prolonged, they wring us dry.

- Poor emotional management patterns, as in frequent outbursts, mean that we use up more energy than others.

- Worry, anxiety, emotional conflict drain Spleen Qi and run us ragged. They tire us out

Wrong treatment including wrong self-treatment

Stimulating or over-draining

- Medications that keep us alert and awake: the drug forces us to perform long after we need rest. Wonderful in emergencies but eventually insidious. Although it feels as if the drug is providing the boost, it is actually our body's reaction to the drug that boosts us, and the energy for this comes from our Yin resources. Often we use, in Western medical parlance, our adrenal gland resources, though Yin deficiency goes beyond just adrenal insufficiency.

- Bleeding obviously reduces our blood reserves. It takes time and energy to replace these and if, forced by circumstances, we have to continue working, we draw heavily on Yin reserves.

- Blood-letting or leeching[8]: both have a long and honourable history but over-use by European doctors who did not understand the underlying principle killed so many patients that the therapy fell out of use. Over-use, like heavy bleeding, drains the body.

- Cupping[9] too frequently. Cupping is a wonderful therapy, practised worldwide for thousands of years, from Europe to China. A cup with hot air is placed upside down on the skin: as the air cools it draws the flesh up into the vacuum. In Chinese medicine terms, it moves blood. But too much cupping can be enervating, reducing our reserves.

- Acupuncture[10]. You might think that acupuncture could do not harm. Indeed, even inappropriate acupuncture is often soon stabilised by the body's natural metabolism. But not always. For example, over-stimulation of acupuncture points can dissipate the body's energy and, since acupuncture points influence the body's metabolism, can weaken it.

8. http://www.acupuncture-points.org/blood-stasis.html
9. http://www.acupuncture-points.org/cupping.html
10. http://www.acupuncture-points.org/acupuncture-theory.html

Someone rang me for help because ever since having had frequent, strong electro-acupuncture, his nervous system had been disrupted, he had become forgetful, tremulous, exhausted, unable to sleep properly, and quite unable to concentrate. There was some sweating at night and continuing pain round where the needles had been inserted. Not surprisingly he was most reluctant to have more acupuncture. His symptoms suggested a considerable element of Yin deficiency.

- X-ray. Radiological scans including MRI, PET and CT scans are, in Chinese medicine, potentially *heating* and *drying*. If aimed to kill tumours, the intention may justify the means, but in Chinese medicine they also disrupt Yin-moistening and nourishing processes. This can lead to Yin deficiency symptoms. Very high intensity X-rays or similar can literally burn us up, quickly consuming all our supplies of fluids and even bone life.

- Primary and secondary effects. Modern medicine has saved many lives and removed much pain and misery. As experience shows, many new drugs have secondary, unwanted effects. The Primary effect of the medication is to suppress unwanted signs or symptoms of disease. The Secondary effect is the body's reaction, often suppressed by more medication. So a drug for headache may quell the main bad headache but produce another kind of headache. Indeed, secondary effects often lead to the withdrawal of the drug by the manufacturer. This may be because the individuals tested during development of the drug may not have represented a sufficiently wide sample of the population, or may not have been healthy. Testing drugs on people with a disease may produce radically different results from testing the drug on healthy people. The latter show you primarily the secondary effects of the medication. Testing the drug on the kind of ill people the drug is aimed at shows mainly, or at least initially, just the Primary effect of the drug[11].

- Drugs, social. These are mainly aimed at raising or loosening the mood. Some of them give you a 'high'. That 'high' comes at a price which is depletion of Yin. The younger you are, assuming maturity, the more often you can partake, but eventually continued exposure to the drug will produce Yin deficiency symptoms. If you become addicted, withdrawal often demonstrates symptoms of Blood and/or Yin deficiency, with shaking, mild fever, loss of skin and eye lustre, lack of will-power, anger, petulance, attention-seeking behaviour, undernourishment and so on.

- Herbs. If drugs are like concentrated herbs, herbs are like concentrated foods, but without the nutrition. They work through the digestion and unless balanced by other herbs may weaken it. Herbs that are too *spicy* may destroy Stomach *Yin*[12]. Herbs that are too *cold* may weaken Spleen *Yang*[13]. In both cases, nutrient absorption is compromised, depleting Blood, which is itself a form or Yin.

- Manipulation, too frequent: this affects the body's structure, especially the tendons holding bones in place. After it, people feel more relaxed and in less pain. But the body is not fooled for very long and often produces other symptoms

11. http://www.acupuncture-points.org/primary-and-secondary-actions.html
12. http://www.acupuncture-points.org/stomach-yin-deficiency.html
13. http://www.acupuncture-points.org/spleen-yang.html

that may be unrecognised as relating to the original manipulation.

For example, an old man sought treatment for knee pain. After a few treatments by manipulation, the knee pain ceased, or at least he stopped complaining of it, but he began to say that his hips hurt. With further manipulation these also improved, in time, but then he began getting severe tension in his upper back, worsening as the hip pain reduced. This stopped him sleeping and made him even more irascible. He did not see this progression, from the extremities towards the centre, as positive so he stopped manipulation and came for acupuncture. This gradually eased the back and hip pains, until the knee pain returned. This eventually cleared with sophisticated acupuncture channel treatment.

- Massage, too deep or frequent. For some people regular massage is irreplaceable and highly beneficial. Done too strongly, too often, however, and it becomes weakening, being almost like a shock to the system. This depletes Yin.

Nutrition[14]

- 'Irregular' eating patterns. As you'll see in the list below, this covers more than just not eating enough. Long-term, poor nutrition is one of the surest and most insidious ways to deplete Yin. At any one time the adverse result is negligible, but over time the body does not absorb what it needs.

14. http://www.acupuncture-points.org/nutrition.html

Instead it draws on its Yin resources, depleting them instead. Poor nutrition means that they are not replenished. Irregular eating includes

- eating while working
- eating at irregular times
- eating too fast
- not chewing
- poor choice of foods
- fast foods
- eating when also drinking alcohol in quantity
- eating when exhausted
- eating while exercising
- not resting after meals

Of course, our bodies have certainly evolved to be able to cope with these bad habits from time to time, but not on an ongoing basis. Some of the above are expanded upon below.

- Foods that over-stimulate eg coffee[15], spicy food, sweets: these make us burn energy but fail to provide us with compensating nutrition. Our bodies react to them by producing a spurt of Yang energy, drawing on Yin reserves to do so. When you are young, your Yin reserves are plentiful and fairly easy to regenerate. As you age, or after illness or one of the other causes mentioned in this chapter, your Yin resources and your ability to regenerate them both diminish.

- However, the power of caffeine, and similar drugs is such that they force your body to perform at a higher intensity, so for a while, you feel wonderful, energised and positive. Once

15. http://www.acupuncture-points.org/coffee.html

the Yang effect has worn off, usually after about 4 hours, you feel low-spirited and exhausted.

I once had a patient who wanted treatment to stop smoking. She smoked about 60 cigarettes daily and it transpired that most of these were when drinking coffee. A university professor, she needed funding for her department. That funding only came if they produced high-quality research documents. The pressure on her to produce these and to apply for grants for research meant that she needed to work at great intensity for 18 hours or more daily. To maintain this level of intensity she took strong coffee almost continuously. However, coffee increased her heart-beat and made her perspire: it also made her jumpy and nervous and she reported that she slept poorly, often waking in a sweat. (She was nowhere near her menopause.) So she smoked tobacco to calm herself down. She was thin, and reported that although she ate well, she was gaining no weight despite taking no exercise: indeed, she thought her weight might have reduced a bit in the year since she took up her appointment.

Here was a situation where one drug (tobacco) was suppressing some of the symptoms caused by another drug, (caffeine). She said that if she stopped the coffee, she had no energy and couldn't work. So she took it and kept on a kind of 'high'. Caffeine was draining her Yin resources, evidenced by the perspiration, insomnia, exhaustion when she stopped it, probable weight loss and nerviness. She was one of only a few clients whom I was unable to help stop smoking, because her need for it remained too high whilst she continued to take coffee.

- As listed above – poor choice of food. Some foods, like

refined and sweetened foods, or those with preservatives, herbicides, flavourings and colourings, take almost as much energy to digest as they give us, or they may give us calories but they lack vitamins and minerals and indeed may deplete our supplies of these, leeching them from our bones.

- Food lacking nutritive quality[16]. Intensive farming has depleted the mineral content of our soils[17]. Without fertilisers, pesticides and herbicides, the plants die. When we eat them they are a poor substitute for the real thing because the plants contain less nutrition than before.

- Alcohol[18] in small quantities seems to harm few people and to relax many. In larger amounts, it has, in Chinese medicine, a heating effect, leading to various kinds of inflammation and eventually, for example, cirrhosis of the liver. On the way there, its heating effect disturbs sleep and often causes sweating. Poor sleep prevents proper recovery, and sweating dissipates fluids. Both predispose to Yin deficiency.

- Poison elicits strong symptoms as the body tries to metabolise, destroy and excrete the poison. Unless you are already Yin deficient, mild poisons cause you few long-term problems and in small quantities may even have a stimulating effect on your metabolism: this is, after all, the basis for homoeopathic philosophy. Large doses of poisons, if not fatal, require a huge effort of your body and can weaken you for a long period. This can drain either Yin and/ or Yang resources.

- Chemicals are added to food to preserve, protect or make it more tasty. They have to be metabolised by our bodies. In the short run, ill-effects would, one might hope, be picked up by manufacturers. Long-term, it is thought that they may

16. See http://www.natural-health-information-centre.com/depleted-soils.html
17. http://www.scientificamerican.com/article/soil-depletion-and-nutrition-loss/
18. http://www.acupuncture-points.org/hangover.html

interfere with food absorption, weakening our ability to
regenerate Yin resources.

- Fasting, starvation. For many people, occasional fasting for
short periods may be beneficial, depending on their
physiology, metabolism and health. Long-term, it means
they take in no nutrients to replace those used in surviving,
so weakening themselves. To keep the body going it draws
on Yin reserves.

- Over-eating: why and how might this drain Yin? Chinese
energy physiology supposes that our digestion needs Yang
energy to be able to process, move and transform food. For
example, Stomach Yang[19] warms food, Spleen Yang[20]
transforms it. That Yang energy comes from Kidney Fire, and
this Fire burns by using our Yin reserves. Gross over-eating
for long periods therefore drains Kidney Fire and Yin. Of
course, on the other side, if the food is highly nutritious,
properly prepared, chewed properly, not difficult to digest
and is given time to digest between meals, Yin will be
replenished by it but in theory, over-eating does eventually
drain Yin. Depending on the food in question and our
metabolism we may or may not put on weight. If the food is
low in nutrition and high in calories, especially if high in
sweet foods, and if we take no exercise, we shall almost
certainly put on weight while, at the same time, eventually
show signs of Yin deficiency.

- Underlying Stomach deficiency. Poor eating habits, especially
if thinking about work while eating, or eating while 'on the
run', or eating when tired or in the late evening, weaken
Stomach Qi. It fails to produce Yin fluids for the body,
depleting Yin reserves. This produces the classic 'Empty Heat'
signs of Yin deficiency, including thirst, not to drink lots but
to drink a little at a time (lots of fluid overwhelms the

19. http://www.acupuncture-points.org/stomach.html
20. http://www.acupuncture-points.org/spleen-yang.html

Stomach); constant appetite but not to eat lots; feeling of mild fever in the afternoon and evening and sweating at night.

- Some thin people who are trying to put on weight and have weak Stomach Qi or lack Kidney Yang[21], eat huge meals, or eat more at a time than they can handle. These overwhelm their Stomach. (If this is the case, after eating they often get eructations, hiccup, burp or get phlegm in their throats or nose, or feel uncomfortably distended or, later, get loose bowel movements showing undigested food. Of course, these symptoms apply to anyone who overwhelms his/her Stomach.)

- Antibiotics are a real hazard for the digestion. In Chinese medicine they are thought to be cooling in their effect, hence their ability to fight inflammatory '*heating*' infections. But they also reduce Stomach Heat or Yang, preventing the digestion from processing food. Often the tongue loses its coating, an indication of Stomach deficiency. Another indication of this cooling effect is runny stools and exhaustion. Unable to digest food properly, the Stomach cannot replenish Yin fluids, weakening Yin reserves.

To replace good ('beneficial') bacteria destroyed by antibiotics, we are often urged to take 'pro-biotics'. These occur in natural, untreated yogurt for example. But yogurt is considered a cold food in Chinese medicine so unless taken with compensating herbs (eg ginger root),

21. http://www.acupuncture-points.org/kidney-yang-deficiency.html

or in the form of dried powder (with warm water) it may increase the cooling effect of the medication, further impeding recovery. Probably just as good as yogurt, however, are fermented foods such as sauerkraut, kimchi, many pickled vegetables, kombucha and miso, most of which are either warming or less cooling than yogurt.

- Too much or too frequent drying or dried food. Dry food requires moisture to digest. That moisture is supplied first by the Stomach, so using up its Yin reserves, and eventually drawing on the body's Yin reserves.

Lack of structure or stability in life, a chaotic lifestyle

- Lack of rest: the 24-hour life leads to a lack of 'downtime'. Probably lack of rest is the single biggest cause of Yin deficiency. Those who have financial resources can enjoy the freedom that a global economy and light 24 hours a day give them. They are fortunate to live in these times. However, without finance, one must work the hours demanded by an employer. But whether or not employed, research[22] on maturing adults between 14 and 22 showed that the more television watched the more problems there were with insomnia.

- Impatience. This may seem a strange cause but nowadays

22. 'NEW STUDY LINKS EXTENSIVE TELEVISION VIEWING IN ADOLESCENCE TO SLEEP PROBLEMS IN EARLY ADULTHOOD' News release from New York State Psychiatric Institute at the Columbia University Medical Center and the Mount Sinai Medical Center 7 June 2004.

we aren't prepared to wait either for things to develop or to buy the latest product. The internet gives us huge advantages but learning to wait is not one of them. We spend less time just enjoying life as nature provides it and we don't like waiting: we think it's wasted time and that we should be busy or at least occupied. Being bored is not an option: we expect our lives to be filled with diversions all the time. This behaviour nurtures a form of anticipatory excitement that eventually drains our yin resources.

- Shift patterns of work. While some people adapt readily to this, others take ages to recover when changing shifts. Short-term this may not matter. Long-term, research shows the damage that shift-work can cause, not least to mental equilibrium.

- Lack of exercise. For most of us, only in the last 200 years have there been jobs where little exercise was required. Until then, if you worked, you exercised, by walking, lifting, carrying etc. By the evening you were physically tired. This exercise forced our bodies to maintain muscle mass, cardiovascular fitness and, given adequate nutrition, a robust immune system. Now we spend so much time sitting that our bodies deteriorate unless we build in exercise. For many, sport compensates, but for everyone else, there is a slow deterioration in fitness and the ability to stay healthy. As is now recognised, insufficient weight-bearing exercise, for example as in walking or standing, allows our bones to deteriorate and develop osteoporosis. Good health, as most people recognise, is the greatest blessing and a superb Yin resource. Lack of exercise dissipates it.

- Too much exercise. Some people exercise too much: to maintain their equilibrium it becomes a necessity. Although exercise is one of the best ways to release tension and stress, too much exhausts us. Occasional exhaustion is no problem: our genes have evolved to deal with it. Continual exhaustion drains us and reduces our immunity. Fit though world athletes are, at their level of training for peak performance, there is a fine line between training within and beyond physical limits. Of course, to get stronger, fitter, faster etc, they push themselves all the time. But if they start getting frequent signs of lowered immunity, of not properly recovering between training sessions, they may be pushing too hard, draining their resources.

- Stress[23]. We are built to manage stress, but we need time to recover. Because the need to keep up with progress and to maintain and improve living standards is forever with us, with stress we feel we can never relax. This puts a huge strain on our Yin resources.

- Worry (finance, relationships, freedom, measured against the norm of society): as with stress, depletes us. In Chinese medicine, worry particularly affects the Spleen energy. The Spleen is central to producing Blood from food, and Blood is central to replenishing Yin supplies.

- Lack of sleep. Good sleep is when our bodies get closest to the vegetative state, the organic process when we repair and replenish supplies. Muscle repair and growth takes place most when our growth hormone somatotropin is released during sleep, particularly during the first, deepest, delta wave sleep of the night. Lack of sleep is one of the greatest inhibitors of growth hormone. Without those repairs, we have to draw on our Yin resources, depleting them.

- Exhaustion. Continued exhaustion means our bodies have no ability to repair ourselves, so have to draw ever deeper on our Yin reserves to survive.

- Sex. Sex has huge psychological and physical benefits for the individual. However, in men, too frequent ejaculation is

23. http://www.acupuncture-points.org/signs-of-stress.html

harmful, lowering energy and spirits. Of course, when fit and young, most men recover almost immediately. However, when ill or older, recovery takes much longer and in Chinese medicine, frequent sex is discouraged for them. Probably having sex too frequently for women is not harmful unless, one supposes it is at such intensity that they are continually exhausted beyond the point of easy recovery. However, for them, having babies too close together, or not taking time to recover properly after giving birth, or when ill, or very heavy menstrual flows are a kind of equivalent: they can drain a woman's resources.

• Sex and drugs. Putting aside the harmful effects of the drugs themselves, the danger of mixing sex and drugs is that drugs enhance sexual desire and may make men, in particular, exhaust themselves faster through over-stimulation and more frequent ejaculation.

EXTERNAL CAUSES

Disease from external pathogenic factors ie virus, bacteria

Every disease absorbs our energy as our body fights it, but our bodies have evolved to deal with this, within limits. The larger our energy output, or the longer it continues, the more energy it takes: intense, especially febrile, disease or prolonged chronic disease both burn up the body's reserves.

Two examples:

A patient brought her son, aged about 9 months. She had eventually realised that he was sensitive to milk and some other foodstuffs but as a result the child was in an advanced state of exhaustion, to the extent that his once strong voice was now weak and he looked exhausted, with black rings under his eyes, poor complexion, tendency to sleep even though his sleep was poor, and so on. With the right treatment he recovered quickly – in fact within just a few days.

A patient of 85, after a successful career in public life, got acute shingles (Herpes simplex) badly. The excruciating pain prevented sleep and any rest and he lost weight, lost energy and lost spirit. He began sweating at unusual times, his back started to hurt and his hearing worsened (these are symptoms of Kidney Yin deficiency[24]). Treatment helped his sleep, reduced the pain and gave him his spirits back, and he was able to start going for walks again, but progress was slow and some pain remained for a long time.

In these examples one sees the disadvantage of old age. The child's powers of recovery produced a quick turnaround, unlike those of the 85 year old.

24. http://www.acupuncture-points.org/kidney-yin-deficiency.html

Electromagnetic influences: X-Rays, wavelengths, mobile phones

The sun can both heat and dry you. Skin exposed to strong sunlight for too long loses its oils, dries and ages faster. However, sunlight increases our body's ability to create Vitamin D, vital for health.

The ideal time-exposure to the sun is when we achieve our best levels of Vitamin D. Of course we want a tan too, and there's the problem – getting the tan takes longer than getting the vitamin D!

Evidence of damage done by mobile phones and the masts carrying their signals is strongly contested. X-Ray damage when concentrated on tissues is used therapeutically, but is regarded as being very heating in Chinese medicine. If those effects are indeed heating, then in theory at least, signals at other electromagnetic wavelengths should also be heating, though perhaps attenuated by distance.

Environment and climate

Pollution, if it drains us faster than our bodies can regenerate their energy, leads to Yin deficiency. Such pollution can be:

• In the air

• From smoking tobacco or other drugs

• Man-made climates

• Heat[25], Cold[26] and Wind[27]: Western medicine sees no problem from heat or wind, but does recognise bacteria and viruses as diseases. The Chinese classification into Heat and Wind merely recognises how they viewed the reactions of the body to such external agents of disease. Make no

25. http://www.acupuncture-points.org/Heat.html
26. http://www.acupuncture-points.org/cold.html
27. http://www.acupuncture-points.org/wind.html

mistake! The ancient Chinese grappled with disease reactions just as severe as anything encountered nowadays, and did so without the benefits of modern pharmacology. It is easy to understand how febrile disease can drain the body but what about Cold?

A 65 year-old patient admits he may have slept poorly for several days before he had an invasion of Cold, so was perhaps more susceptible to it than otherwise. He worked in a cool basement but the room he worked in was warm. However, on the day (mid-winter) in question, the outside door, near the room he worked in, had been removed for repairs. The day got colder quickly and temperatures fell far below freezing by midday. As he was often outside the door to his office, and because he had no extra clothes to wear, he got very cold. Because of appointments, he could not go home early. By early evening he was shivering uncontrollably. Hot drinks were welcome but he felt icy cold. Once home he had a very warm bath but the shivering chill continued even abed with numerous warm bean bags for company. With subsequent treatment his uncontrollable shivering abated but it took him several weeks to feel comfortably warm, with warm hands etc, again. Even after all this, his energy remained sapped until he returned for more treatment. Here was an invasion of Cold, with a strongly energy-sapping effect.

- Fevers are normally part of the body's comprehensive assault on an invading pathogen. Evolution has given us strong powers to defend ourselves. However, beyond a certain point, fevers become a problem. This occurs if the fever cannot kill the pathogen or if it goes on for too long, draining energy.

- Dehydration, whether from fever or lack of moisture or hot weather, is potentially a medical emergency, especially when the brain is affected, when it can lead to symptoms of shock.

One patient was trapped in a railway carriage during a very hot drought. The air-conditioning failed, and for safety reasons passengers were not allowed to leave the train. Water ran out. Passengers took it in turn to lie on the floor, the coolest place. A number of passengers needed some days in hospital following this and my patient was still in a very weakened condition, with peculiar night sweats even during subsequent cold weather, back pain, a tendency to dizziness, strong tinnitus and very low energy levels, when he eventually visited me 6 weeks later.

- Wind symptoms happen fast, and symptoms change quickly. Sudden shivering then hot sweats, sneezing then dry nose, pains that migrate from place to place in the body, are all symptoms of what the Chinese named 'Wind' symptoms. Because they act fast, they do not usually drain Yin energy unless peculiarly intense.

When a Yin depleting factor goes on for too long, the body begins to display signs of heat, partially or wholly. At times the patient will feel cold, but then, more often in the afternoon and evening, feels uncomfortably warm, with warm hands and feet. Here the Yin deficiency has allowed a new syndrome to develop, called 'Empty Heat[28]'. As it proceeds it can become more obvious and more destructive, draining Yin even faster.

However, Yin deficiency can exist for years before Empty Heat appears. On the tongue, Yin deficiency shows as a lack of coating and gradual increase of cracks in the tongue surface. Empty Heat shows, additionally, as a change of colour in the tongue from normal to red, also eventually with cracks.

Yin deficiency mainly affects the Stomach, Lungs, Liver, Heart and Kidney, and sometimes the Spleen energy organs, often in that order.

The symptoms described below for each zang-fu energy organ make more sense when you understand what organ does in Chinese medicine, for which read the pages in the footnotes.

Stomach Yin deficiency

Think of Stomach yin deficiency as being a deficiency in the physical structure and fluids of the stomach. However, as observed in Chinese medicine, following Stomach yin deficiency *physical* symptoms there will eventually also appear *mental* symptoms.

Mentally,

- often brain-fagged
- can't get thoughts together
- rather nervous and
- sensitive to slight causes and worries.

Physically,

- tiredness yet also tension
- digestion is unreliable, with little appetite ...

28. See chapter 8 and http://www.acupuncture-points.org/empty-heat-and-cold.html

- ... or feels full after very little food
- may have mild heartburn
- or a dull pain after food
- Dryness of mucous membranes; mouth, throat, stools
- The pulse is empty and floating[29] in the Stomach position

Stomach Yin deficiency problems arise mostly from

- What Chinese medicine calls an 'irregular diet', which means poor eating habits, including skipping meals, eating always in a hurry or when otherwise occupied, leaving no time to digest food before rushing on to the next job, eating when worrying, etc. For more on this see chapter 9 and the footnote[30].
- Medications such as antibiotics, taken for too long or too often
- Genetic causes, perhaps when parents were also very thin

Lung Yin[31] deficiency

Mentally,

- rather slow and melancholy
- doubting himself
- easily depressed
- often doubts he will ever get better

Physically:

---

29. 'Empty' and 'Floating' are pulse qualities recognised in Chinese medicine. See more about this at http://www.acupuncture-points.org/pulse-diagnosis.html
30. http://www.acupuncture-points.org/nutrition.html
31. http://www.acupuncture-points.org/lung-yin.html

- tendency to catch colds easily
- weak voice, or it lacks endurance and
- he doesn't want to talk
- sweats easily even without exertion
- dislikes and has no resistance to cold, and
- has cold hands and a cold upper back, especially when tired
- Cough: slight, often from talking with ...
- ... lots of watery catarrh
- Very little thirst, and if he drinks, usually prefers warm drinks
- Complexion is pale but often shiny
- Pulse is usually floating and empty[32]; may be fast

Lung Yin problems arise mostly from

- Smoking tobacco over many years, or being exposed to it for long periods, say throughout childhood and teens
- Overuse of the voice, for years, as in the case of actors, sergeant majors, clergymen or speech makers
- Sadness, grief. These emotions can have a major effect on Lung Qi

Liver Yin deficiency

Mentally:

- low spirits
- lack of initiative and tendency to irritability

Physically:

32. These are terms used in pulse diagnosis in Chinese medicine. For more, see http://www.acupuncture-points.org/pulse-diagnosis.html

- Vertigo
- eye problems such as dryness and floaters
- easily tired from eye-strain eg at computers or reading
- tingling in the limbs and numbness
- often cramps, when tired or in bed late in the evening
- Pale face, though cheek bones may be red
- Brittle nails
- Skin dryness
- Poor sleep, often from waking without apparent cause
- Pulse is floating and empty, and a little fast

Liver[33] Yin deficiency problems arise mostly from

- Long-term Emotional exhaustion
- Poor food choices leading to Blood deficiency
- Physical exercise above one's natural levels of attainment
- Heavy blood loss, as during heavy menstruation or from wounds

Heart Yin deficiency

Mentally,

- anxiety which can run away with itself, leading to wild ideas and speculations and easy panic
- At night, sleep can be badly disturbed by dreams
- Hard to concentrate
- Poor memory

33. http://www.acupuncture-points.org/liver-functions.html

- Lacking steadiness
- Easily startled
- Upset even by trifles

Physically,

- Frequent palpitations – the heart can race or bound or pump fiercely, often without reason
- Face can feel flushed
- Mouth and throat often feel dry, more so later in the day and evening
- Pulse is empty and floating and a little rapid

Heart[34] Yin deficiency problems arise mostly from

- Long-term emotional 'exhaustion', as from anxiety or fear
- Exposure to great heat, as from the climate or environment
- Working for too long under stress

Kidney Yin deficiency[35]

Mentally,

- doesn't feel able to work, from weak memory, difficult comprehension and lack of concentration

Physically,

- Dryness of mouth and throat, mainly at night
- Perspiration during sleep at night

---

34. http://www.acupuncture-points.org/heart.html
35. http://www.acupuncture-points.org/kidney-yin.html

- Lumbar weakness and pain, better lying down, though restless
- Urine is dark and scanty
- Often dizzy
- Noises and/or a sense of pressure in his ears, and poor hearing
- Usually constipated
- Lassitude
- Pulse is usually floating and empty and may be a little fast

Spleen Yin deficiency

Mentally,

- Worry
- Over-thinking
- Too much caring for others
- Tendency to obsess

Physically,

- Dry mouth
- Dry throat
- Dry lips
- Thin body
- Weak appetite
- Abdominal distension after eating
- Dry stools
- Dull complexion

- Night-sweating
- Pulse is of thin quality

Spleen[36] Yin problems arise mostly from

- What in Chinese medicine is called an 'irregular diet', meaning bad eating habits, like eating during work or when standing or when driving or worrying about work, or eating at odd times without regularity, gulping food rather than chewing it, and so on (for more on this see chapter 9)[37].
- Over-exertion
- Worry and over-thinking, or over-caring for others

Because the Energy organs are all connected, Yin deficiency in one of them can spread to another. For example, Liver Yin deficiency can 'spread' to Kidney Yin[38] and Heart Yin deficiencies. With Liver Yin deficiency it is not uncommon to see the development of Liver Yang excess[39] patterns.

36. For more on Spleen energy problems see http://www.acupuncture-points.org/spleen.html
37. See also http://www.acupuncture-points.org/nutrition.html
38. See http://www.acupuncture-points.org/liver-and-kidney-yin-deficiency.html
39. See http://www.acupuncture-points.org/liver-yang.html

CHAPTER 5

Mental Symptoms of Yin Deficiency

This chapter emphasises mental symptoms but contains some physical symptoms. In Chinese medicine they are not separated, just different places on a continuum.

As Chapter 4, (the Causes of Yin deficiency) explained, for most people Yin deficiency appears slowly, the main exceptions being after a very high fever or exposure to extreme heat or heating rays when, after the heat reaction has died down, the body's supply of Yin fluids has been consumed and exhausted.

Consequently, most people hardly notice as their Yin deficiency develops. As people age, other illness-conditions appear, such as more frequent colds and coughs, stiff joints, skin eruptions, noises in the ears after drinking too much coffee and so on. While these are noticed, any accompanying or underlying Yin deficiency is overlooked.

So as our Yin deficiency gradually emerges, what symptoms might we attribute to it?

Bear in mind that Yin and Yang, for health, should balance one another so that any temporary increase or decrease in one or other is quickly brought back into balance.

Yin is stabilising, calming, steadying, nourishing and supporting. Without it, what happens?

There is a spectrum between restlessness and internal heat. Internal – 'Empty' – Heat is sensed almost like a fever, and sometimes does produce a low fever, but commonly just makes you feel uncomfortably warm – often unexpectedly – although in time you begin to realise that these symptoms are usually worse in the late afternoon and evening.

Restlessness of mind is harder to deal with. The mind seems always active. At the time people don't regard this as a problem and it may even seem enjoyable. The problem comes from never stopping to rest, even though exhausted.

Although the following lists of symptoms and those in the next chapter on Physical symptoms can seem long, you do not have to have all the symptoms listed to qualify for Yin Deficiency!

To be diagnosed you need a few of them but an acupuncturist would probably decide for sure after talking to you, viewing your tongue[1] and assessing your pulse[2].

- With Mind always active, they cannot concentrate for long, and memory weakens

- This excess thinking is very hard to switch off

- This makes them anxious

- They become moody, nervous and, to friends, seem ungrounded

- Sleep becomes a problem, either in getting off to sleep or from frequent waking, or from very light sleep, so that they seldom feel they have had a restorative rest

- They can become impulsive, hurried and sometimes impetuous, but with it, unsure of themselves

1. http://www.acupuncture-points.org/tongue-diagnosis.html
2. http://www.acupuncture-points.org/pulse-diagnosis.html

- Temper can become irascible, moods unreliable
- They can become agitated, aggressive, hasty and over-reactive
- To slights they become ultra-sensitive, then make it worse by worrying
- They may seem interested in everything, only because they ...
- ... lack the mental energy to concentrate on just one thing
- Sometimes they have a big appetite, never assuaged
- Some, as their condition begins to develop, can even seem loud, noisy people until their deeper fears are exposed, when all the puff goes out of them
- Inside, they are often burning up mentally, with inexplicable fears and imaginings
- Some people can display signs of obsessive compulsion
- Yin deficiency symptoms appear in many forms of Western Mental disease – see chapter 3. Although Chinese medicine is not a universal panacea, treating people for Yin deficiency often does help their mental condition to improve
- NB Some of the more extreme symptoms mentioned begin to spread from Yin deficiency into other syndromes

PTSD Post Traumatic Stress Syndrome

Syndromes now recognised as post-traumatic stress syndrome often show strong symptoms of Yin deficiency. The shock cripples them and they need care, often institutional care or care at home, to give them time to recover.

They may show signs of both Yin and/or Yang deficiency. Like nearly everyone, they recover faster from Yang deficiency[3] than

3. http://www.acupuncture-points.org/yang-deficiency.html

from Yin deficiency although with appropriate treatment young people can recover faster from the latter than expected.

ADHD Attention Deficit Hyperactive Disorder

In Chinese medicine, ADHD can be due to several syndromes. The Yin deficient form has the typical dryness (of mouth, for example), night sweats, ear noises, sleeplessness and poor memory alongside the inability to concentrate.

Another form, with daydreaming, slowness and vagueness, has been described as a state of inattention from brains that are subject to *theta* wave patterns more than *beta* and *alpha* wave patterns. Theta patterns occur naturally at medium depths of sleep.

A curious thing is that these levels are sometimes reached by intense meditators who can maintain these mental rhythms even though fully awake and aware: perhaps this explains why they float through life in a wonderfully unstressed way – but of course this mental state has been attained after considerable practice, effort and time.

Not so for this kind of ADHD sufferer, who appears to lack consolidating mechanisms, possibly attributable to poor nutrition or genes. At any rate, this form of ADHD is probably closer to *Spleen and Heart Qi and/or Blood deficiency*[4] than to Yin deficiency in general.

---

4. http://www.acupuncture-points.org/heart-and-spleen-blood-deficiency.html . This may eventually lead to symptoms of http://www.acupuncture-points.org/heart-and-kidney-yin-deficiency-with-empty-heat.html

In writing this paragraph, I take a risk! Be aware that what I say is speculative!

In looking for the causes of ADHD which I saw no signs of when at school and university in the 1950s and 1960s, I suggest that there may be an elephant in the room which nobody likes to mention.

This is the intense programme of *immunisation* given to children under the age of two. While there is little doubt that immunisations have helped to reduce the incidence of many diseases, forcing them on children before their immune systems have had time to develop (indeed, giving them then partly *because* of that) may be weakening their resources at a very early stage, making them more susceptible to hyperactivity later because they lack effective or strong yin stabilising resources.

This is a huge and contentious subject but it is noteworthy that some yin-enhancing nutritional approaches to ADHD and similar conditions have often been at least partially effective, particularly those that reduce yang foods (such as junk, sugary and spicy foods) and increase yin foods (such as appropriate oils, eg omega 3-rich fish oil).

The following pages on my website explore this in different ways:

- http://www.acupuncture-points.org/suppression.html
- http://www.acupuncture-points.org/lung-qi-deficiency.html
- http://www.acupuncture-points.org/disease-process.html
- http://www.acupuncture-points.org/remaining-pathogenic-factor.html

- http://www.acupuncture-points.org/nutritive-and-defensive-qi-disharmony.html

- http://www.acupuncture-points.org/chronic-fatigue-syndrome-acupuncture.html

- http://www.acupuncture-points.org/homeopathic-remedy.html

Manic depression – bipolar disorder – which you might think was at one end due to Yang deficiency and at the other to Yang excess, is actually diagnosed usually as an alternation between Yin excess, in the form of Damp[5] and Phlegm[6] clouding the mind and dulling the energy, and Yang excess[7], in the form of Fire[8].

However, if this form of Yang excess continues for too long, it can consume Yin, leading to Yin deficiency as well.

In Chinese medicine, Yin deficiency mental symptoms are classified according to the Energy Organ (the technical term is Zang-fu[9]) involved. By so classifying the kind of Yin deficiency, treatment can be directed more specifically with faster results.

However, bear in mind that just as Yin deficiency usually takes time to appear, treatment to get rid of it also takes time and works better when the patient makes changes. In fact, most

5. http://www.acupuncture-points.org/damp.html
6. http://www.acupuncture-points.org/phlegm.html
7. http://www.acupuncture-points.org/yang-excess.html
8. http://www.acupuncture-points.org/fire.html
9. http://www.acupuncture-points.org/zang-fu.html

experienced practitioners agree that if the patient makes no change in lifestyle and diet, improvement will be impossible, or very short-lived.

As Yin deficiency develops, there may in time also arrive what is called Empty Heat[10]. This may not appear for many years, but can appear within weeks, depending on the strength of the underlying constitution and its susceptibility.

Empty Heat is more unsettling because it produces a sensation of heat, of flushing, intolerance of warmth or warm clothing (often only temporary because they cool quickly when the skin is exposed to cool air), greater thirst and dryness, the symptoms often worsening from mid-afternoon onwards.

This heat can be felt not just in the mouth and throat but also in the ears and on the face, making the cheekbones look pink – even 'healthy' to some eyes, unfortunately.

With Empty Heat, irritability occurs faster and anxiety is greater.

Depending on which Energy organ is most affected, there may be:

- **Kidney Yin** deficiency with Empty Heat: Waking at night, with sweating or nocturnal emissions and dreams. There may also be dizziness and ear noises (tinnitus), temporary lapses of concentration and memory. The usual cause is overwork, irregular diet and sometimes some kind of shock or guilt pattern This can lead on to a noticeable lack of determination and will-power, and subsequently to a kind of fearful depression. Very anxious. These symptoms can contribute to the miseries of menopausal flushes. Palms, soles and centre of chest feel uncomfortably warm, worse as the afternoon and evening progress. Ears burn. Cheekbones flush easily or may always be pink. Thirsty, but only for small amounts at a time. Whilst more common in thin people this can affect people who are obese. With Yin deficiency the

10. For more on this, see http://www.acupuncture-points.org/empty-heat-and-cold.html

tongue nearly always lacks a coating: additionally, with Empty Heat the tongue[11] is red.

- **Heart Yin** deficiency with Empty Heat: sleep is very disturbed by dreams, with much insomnia; not only is it hard to get to sleep but you keep waking up. In the chest there are palpitations (by which is meant that you can feel the heart beating when normally you would not, whether or not it is racing or fluttering or bumping); memory is very poor, great anxiety and restlessness, always feeling they should be doing something else, as if uneasy with life; very easily startled. This pattern is more common in older people and comes on with or following Kidney Yin deficiency. With Empty Heat there is also a cheekbone flush with a sensation of increased heat in the afternoon and evening, either on the face, the ears or the mouth and throat.; palms, soles and centre of chest often feel uncomfortably warm; pulse is fast. Thirst for small amounts only. With Yin deficiency the tongue nearly always lacks a coating: additionally, with Empty Heat the tongue becomes red.

- **Liver Yin** deficiency with Empty Heat: depression and dizziness combine, with a sense of aimless restlessness. Insomnia is common, with waking for several hours often after the first two hours of sleep; vision blurred, limbs often feel tingly, numb or as if insects are crawling on them. Underlying this pattern is often stress and an irregular diet (see chapter 9). The stress is not always unpleasant, in fact it may be enjoyed! It could arise from being 'stretched' at work all the time, or with too many jobs or occupations each of which makes great demands. Sometimes this condition arises after pushing oneself too hard physically, and is seen in athletes. However, it can be seen in otherwise ordinary people who expect too much of their bodies: for instance, men who try to achieve huge muscular gains at the

11. http://www.acupuncture-points.org/tongue-diagnosis.html

gym too fast, or women who eat too little and try to lose weight via cardiovascular exercise too quickly. Empty Heat adds the cheekbone flush, general sensation of warmth towards evening, night sweats which are very draining, a sensation of warmth in the chest, palms and soles and sometimes eyes, (which contributes to dryness there and, if the diet is wrong, to symptoms like blepharitis), thirst only for small amounts, and great anxiety. With Yin deficiency the tongue nearly always lacks a coating: additionally, with Empty Heat the tongue is red.

- **Lung Yin** deficiency with Empty Heat: the main mental symptoms of Lung Yin deficiency are a lack of energy which can be experienced as a mild form of depression, and this can manifest as a dislike of talking, or inability to talk for long because the voice runs out of energy or becomes hoarse. The background to this, unless from a chest disease or fever, is often a long period of grief or great sadness. Bad posture, such as leaning over a desk for years, contributes to this. People who speak loudly all the time or have to shout a lot can also develop this. There are usually other physical symptoms, for more of which see Chapter 6, such as dryness of the throat and mouth and frequently a ticklish cough worsened by talking. With Empty Heat, you get also a sensation of warmth, (even mild fever) in the afternoon or evening, often felt in the palms or soles but often mainly in the chest. Thirst increases but only for small amounts at a time. Cheekbones often redder than the rest of the face which may be pale. With Yin deficiency the tongue nearly always lacks a coating: additionally, with Empty Heat the tongue is red.

Bit of technical stuff: Yin deficiency includes Blood deficiency (but not vice versa). This means that, very often, treatment for Yin deficiency also requires more specific treatment for Blood deficiency. In chapter 9 on Nutrition, various foods are described that benefit Blood rather than Yin: as a secondary effect many also benefit Yin.

CHAPTER 6

Physical Symptoms of Yin Deficiency

NB Please don't diagnose yourself based solely on information here. Yin deficiency nearly always develops over time and can initially be hard to recognise. Many of the following symptoms, on their own, also have other explanations.

Some of these symptoms include signs of Yin deficiency with Empty Heat[1], which tends to occur in time after Yin deficiency has taken hold.

By taking precautions as explained later, including changes in lifestyle and diet, we may prevent deterioration, so not notice the symptoms of Yin deficiency for longer, if ever.

Lack of Fluids including of Blood

- Dryness – skin, eyes, lips, mouth, throat , worse at night

- Dryness, hair

- Voice changes, throat and mouth dry

- Floaters – eyes: eye dryness

- Eyes lose ability to see properly: retina deteriorates, lens thickens

1. For more on this, see http://www.acupuncture-points.org/emptyheat-and-cold.html

- Scanty menses
- Urine Scanty and Dark
- Dryness – vagina
- Bloodless – infertility
- Dizziness
- Thirst, usually for cool water, in small sips

Lack of Nourishment

- May have increased appetite, or eats continually
- Muscles don't develop or their mass declines
- Taut tendons, cramps
- Unhealthy skin
- Inability to gain weight
- Loss of weight
- Emaciation, thinness

Lack of Steadiness

- Heart beat – palpitations, irregular: nervousness, over-reaction to stimuli
- Restlessness
- Joints crack
- Bones lose mass – osteoporosis
- Tendency to fall from lack of attention or dizziness

Lack of Coolness – as Empty Heat develops

- Exposes or uncovers feet at night in bed or likes walking barefoot on cold floor

- Burning ears or head
- Warm hands (palms), feet (soles) and chest, worse pm
- Heat and hot flushes/flashes
- Unexpected Sweating, can be drenching, usually at night
- Intolerance of Warmth and Heat
- Mild, sensation of warmth or fever, usually starting during the afternoon and worsening through the evening
- Stronger heat in afternoon, esp palms, soles and chest
- Malar flush (ie cheekbones can look pink) when rest of face remains sallow
- Chronic inflammations eg ongoing sore throat, anus, lungs (cough)
- Chronic urogenital inflammation or low-grade infection
- Skin inflammation, eczema
- Wounds heal only slowly

Lack of Structure, anchoring and routine

- Insomnia with desire to sleep
- Hypertension
- Weakness in core supportive structure, eg bones, knees, back, abdomen
- Desire to lie down, to rest, but restlessness intervenes, or desire to be busy prevents it
- Premature ejaculation
- Tendency to diabetes
- Tendency to stroke
- Insomnia, or sleeping in daytime (not due to shift patterns)

or inability to get to sleep until dawn or very late in night
ie 5am or later

Kidney deficiency symptoms – *which nearly always appear as Yin deficiency develops*

- Back – lumbar pain: eventually may lead to shoulder tension
- Knee problems and weakness
- Legs weak or unsteady
- Ears – hearing deteriorates, tinnitus
- Lack of concentration, and lapses in memory

Tongue[2]

- Lacks a secure, grounded coating but has normal colour
- May be cracked: cracks in new places suggest possible Yin deficiency in the correlated Zang-fu Energy organ. For example, if new cracks appear in the area towards the front of the tongue, they may suggest growing Yin deficiency in the Lungs which are represented by this tongue area
- As Empty Heat develops the tongue's body colour becomes redder but in the early stages, before Empty Heat appears, it may have normal colour
- If Empty Heat appears too, the tongue will feel dry

Pulse[3]

- Floating* – ie not deep: easy to feel under slight touch
- Empty*: lacks resilience
- Faster than normal ('rapid') as Empty Heat develops

2. http://www.acupuncture-points.org/tongue-diagnosis.html
3. http://www.acupuncture-points.org/pulse-diagnosis.html

*'Floating' and 'Empty' are two of some 30 different pulse qualities commonly recognised by acupuncturists trained in Traditional Chinese medicine.

CHAPTER 7

Different Stages of Life

Your inherited constitution, already mentioned in chapter 4, can be hugely important in your life, not least as to if and when you develop Yin deficiency. However, the love, nourishment, support, discipline and education that a child receives as it matures can equally affect how inherited health turns out.

Premature birth: babies born prematurely have lacked the full 38 weeks of nutrition and rest so are almost certainly born with a predisposition to both Blood and Yin deficiency. However, typical Yin deficient signs might not be present at birth. More likely, there will be early signs of Empty Heat[1], appearing as rashes or inflammation (eg in the mouth on the gums when teething) being easily startled, difficulty sleeping, dryness and thirst.

When Chinese medicine first developed, premature birth probably meant an early death, so perhaps they lacked experience of its health implications.

Childhood fevers are common and may be even beneficial unless the fever is extreme or prolonged, when it severely exhausts the body's reserves, leading to potential or real Yin deficiency.

Growing too fast, physically or mentally: sometimes the

1. http://www.acupuncture-points.org/empty-heat-and-cold.html

growth outstrips the supply of healthy nutrition to sustain it. At this point, the body draws heavily on Jing essence[2] to plug the gaps, leading to a tendency to Yin deficiency.

Teens, late nights and lack of sleep, infections. The main problem here is the lack of rest, including sleep. These are years of experimentation and border-exploration. They often mean frequent tiredness. Infection during these years, often intense, and sometimes exhausting, as with post-viral conditions and glandular fever – infectious mononucleosis – drains when energy is most needed.

20s – 40s: lack of sleep, overwork, rearing children, ongoing exhaustion. If the teenage years were those of exploration, this period is often the first when people are tested by work. Careers are forged, success is needed, work hours may be long. At the same time, these are the years when families are started, with interrupted sleep and continual exhaustion.

Too many babies, close together, without proper regeneration of strength between them can weaken or drain a woman's Jing resources. To preserve her career, a woman may rush back to work earlier than is good for either her or her baby's health. If the child misses her badly, this may lead to exhausting psychological demands on her, the family and society later.

Drug culture, never resting, over-activity Social drugs give us not just artificial 'highs' but also the ability to maintain high output for longer. Although the drug stimulates this, it is our bodies which supply the energy.

The culture of 24 hour partying is severely draining of Yin energies.

Too much sex. Although this can apply to women, when it usually happens by starting to child-bear too early or by abuse, leading to sexually transmitted disease and humiliation,

2. http://www.acupuncture-points.org/jing-essence.html

reducing her self-confidence and self-respect, too much sex applies more to men.

This is because ejaculation disperses sperm (as Nature intends) but it also dissipates it. Manufacturing sperm uses Jing essence, which, while available in bountiful quantities in youth, does reduce with age. Men typically go to sleep after sex, to recover. If they don't, or they have, for their particular individual physiology, too much sex, then their Yin resources may become diminished.

Too little sex. In either gender, depending on health, genetics, social norms and physiology, too little sex can be mentally very disturbing, leading to restlessness, tension, anxiety and confidence issues. These emotions can prevent proper rest. In extreme situations that can in turn lead to Yin deficiency.

Anger issues. Constant emotional tension, especially from anger and frustration, drain Yin energy.

Menopause (although there are other syndromes in Chinese medicine besides Yin deficiency which cause menopausal problems). At this time of life, Blood flow to the womb reduces and the woman's endocrine system goes through a major change.

As a result she may suffer from vaginal dryness, skin impoverishment, hair loss, memory lapses, voice changes, insomnia and other symptoms of Blood and Yin deficiency. In some women some of these signs continue indefinitely.

Long-term tiredness or disease. At any age, chronic disease is draining and after it, convalescence may be vital to stop Yin deficiency developing.

Age brings an array of symptoms. Some occur due to Blood not circulating[3], others to lack of nutrition, some to Yin deficiency. People become more prone to insomnia and

3. http://www.acupuncture-points.org/blood-stasis.html

opportune infections, or to the emergence of dormant infections like herpes zoster.

Ageing issues connected with or showing signs of Yin deficiency as the fabric of the body begins to fray include:

- Hair: loses vibrancy, colour and falls out
- Teeth lose resilience, crack, are ground, wear away
- Gums recede; roots weaken
- Hearing diminishes and tinnitus begins
- Bones thin, crack, break
- Joints lose flexibility
- Memory weakens
- Flesh shrivels, dries
- Inter-vertebral discs narrow, height is lost
- Vision becomes less acute, macular degeneration
- Body repairs itself more slowly

Yin Deficiency can be slow to develop

Yin deficiency can exist for years without much of a sign other than lack of coating on the tongue or easy exhaustion and sometimes even these are not obvious. It often combines with other syndromes – for example Qi[4] (Energy) deficiency – which shows up as an increase of
Damp or Phlegm, because the body cannot so easily clear them.

Damp[5] and Phlegm[6] are Yin excess[7] symptoms when, for example, the tongue may be swollen with a white or greasy coating, quite different from the 'classical' Yin deficient tongue which has no coating and, if Empty Heat arises, becomes red.

4. http://www.acupuncture-points.org/qi.html
5. http://www.acupuncture-points.org/damp.html
6. http://www.acupuncture-points.org/phlegm.html
7. http://www.acupuncture-points.org/yin-excess.html

One day some small inflammation may appear that becomes chronic. For example a throat infection continues after a cold or a cough has finished. The mouth and throat are always a little dry, with an occasional ticklish cough. Sometimes the patient wakes in the night with a drenching sweat, for no obvious reason.

As time goes by, the voice becomes a little weak and the individual pushes it a bit harder, making it hoarse. Low energy and the cough take the patient to his doctor who, after tests, finds nothing much wrong. In resignation he prescribes an antibiotic or, better, some rest and improved nourishment – but usually the patient wants the doctor to prescribe.

Antibiotics[8] have a cooling effect (in Chinese medicine) so the throat feels less inflamed for a while. However, unfortunately, side-effects of antibiotics include weakening of the digestion (in Chinese medicine antibiotics usually weaken the Spleen[9] energy). This reduces the nourishment the patient gets from food so he becomes more susceptible to another infection and subsequent inflammation.

With a weak Spleen energy, the patient's body is less able to clear Damp and Phlegm, which swell the tongue and in some circumstances might even mask Yin deficiency. These syndromes thrive on Yin deficiency like weeds in bad soil. The earlier they are sorted out, the better, because as Yin deficiency develops it becomes harder to shift.

8. http://www.acupuncture-points.org/antibiotics.html
9. http://www.acupuncture-points.org/spleen.html

CHAPTER 8

Understanding how to treat Yin Deficiency

In Chinese medicine the 'Principle' of treatment is to

- clear any Empty Heat and then
- nourish Yin

The aim is to stabilise life, to enable the body to catch up with lost sleep and repair of tissues and processes. In addition, it may be necessary to 'pacify Yang and nourish Blood'.

How to understand the need to clear Empty Heat?

Think about a meal you have been cooking on the stove which is now threatening to turn into charcoal as it boils nearly dry. Here, the lack of moisture is the Yin deficiency and the over-heating and potential turning to charcoal is the 'Empty Heat'. If you were to add water the danger would be averted (although this might change the taste).

So, what would you do here? If it was me, I would first remove the pan from the fire – from the heat. Only then would I add, slowly, water. (If you say you would just add water straight away, I would suggest you do more cooking, because, at least in my experience, if you add water to an over-heated dried-out pan, you get a lot of steam and any food remaining boils over and out of the pot!)

Actually this is not a perfect analogy because the heat comes from the stove whereas in real Empty Heat the heat is engendered from within the body not from outside it. (*Your* body is alive, whereas the stove needs you and fuel to come alive.)

This is more akin to a woman returning home after work, hungry and exhausted, to take over minding her children from a childminder. By late afternoon her children are tired, hungry and fractious. For her, this is an added strain. Not uncommonly she is easily irritated and some women get absolutely desperate, nearly apoplectic. Some go red in the face and end up with severe headaches. Many get very hot. Here the heat comes from (yin) exhaustion. Had she been rested and fresh, there might have been no problem.

Amazingly, responsibility and love win out and she manages to restrain herself from violence – but it can be a near thing. That anger can become habitual so that the sight of her children pushes up her blood pressure and a sense of desperation pervades her life.

These sources of apparent Yang come not from external sources such as a bug or a huge flaming row at work, but from exhaustion. Had she not been hungry and tired-out on her return she might have handled her children easily but the deficiencies in her energy and resources led to her frustration, tension, heat and headache.

There can come a point where that internal anger begins to take over and she gets a sense of pressure or heat in her ears and tension in her shoulders all the time, perhaps with palpitations and perspiration, depending on her particular constitutional makeup.

At that point the internal deficiency can move towards

internal 'Heat' as 'pressure' builds up. Typical symptoms of Empty Heat include –

- a sense of heat in palms, soles and central chest;
- sweating at night during sleep when there is no reason for it;
- a sense of heat in the afternoon and evening, (which may be felt all over, or on the face or in the head or ears); sometimes this amounts to a low-grade fever as well, which if you visit your doctor in the afternoon may incline him to think you have an infection;
- A flush over the cheekbones (malar bones) but not elsewhere on the face;
- Sleep disturbed by frequently waking up for short periods;
- A sense of anxiety but often without any reason for it;
- Restlessness: the feeling that you should be doing something;
- Eyelid often has a thin red line inside it;
- Stools tend to be dry, but without pain in the abdomen;
- Sometimes there is mild tinnitus, worse in the evening;
- Skin eruptions, if they occur, are dark red and not raised;
- Tongue has little or no coating and is red and may be peeled;
- Pulse is what is called empty and floating, and faster than usual.
- Other symptoms occur as well, but depend on the particular zang-fu[1] Energy Organ that is affected. Hypertension is common.

You can have Empty Heat with only one or two of these symptoms.

1. http://www.acupuncture-points.org/zang-fu.html

Acupuncture theory suggests that merely treating Yin deficiency here will work only slowly, if at all. The first treatments should be mainly directed at helping to quell the internal 'Empty' Yang Heat[2]. Once she is cooler and calmer, more relaxed, treatments for Yin deficiency will become much more effective.

To work on YOU, treatment also needs YOUR active participation!

- **Time**. Sometimes, in learning to deal with your tendency to Yin deficiency, the best thing you can do is learn to enjoy a slower pace, and sometimes to be bored. Actually, once you have learned to be bored, you may find the world an even more interesting place than before as your senses appreciate a greater awareness of your surroundings.

- **Space**. If you make regular journeys by train or bus, try looking out of the window instead of burying your head in a book, your Kindle, or keeping up with emails. You are likely to be around for less than 100 years and the world, one hopes, will outlast you. There is, still, plenty of space in it for most of us. It's here to live in. Try not to live purely in your head: instead learn to appreciate the sound of birdsong, the feel of a breeze on your skin, the rustle of wind in leaves, the sensation on bare feet of walking on grass: the texture of things.

- **Stability**. If you suffer from Yin deficiency you probably already lack stability. You may need someone else to calm and steady you, perhaps your family, or an institution such as the health service, or a counsellor or group of stable friends. Stability also comes from gardening,

2. Why is it called 'Empty' Yang? This is because it arises from deficient Yin, not from Full or Excess Yang, for which see http://www.acupuncture-points.org/yang-excess.html

or from working on a community project. Joining classes or groups to sing works for many. All are Yin-type resources.

- **Rest**. To start with, you may need to set an alarm clock to tell you when and how often to rest! Just lie down! The floor will do, so long as it is not concrete and you can make it comfortable and warm. But regular rests are a must.

- **Avoidance of stress and learning how to deal with it**, (so watch no horror movies!)

- **Steadying, reliable habits** such as:

- *time to rest during the day;*

- *early bed and extended sleep or occasional naps during the day;*

- *steady work patterns;*

- *relaxed walks preferably in the country;*

- *gardening;*

- *learning to appreciate slow, quiet music, much of which was written between 1600 and 1920 AD;*

- *proper Nutrition (next chapter);*

- *good eating habits;*

- *relaxed, unhurried meals alone or with friends;*

- *learning how to steady the mind (see 'sending Qi downwards', below).*

- **Avoidance of whatever over-stimulates or heats or dries** – ideas, drugs, foods, actions, texting, internet, twitter, 24-hour lifestyle, reading or watching thrillers or exciting ideas or fiction before bedtime. If it tends to keep you 'wired', then it's not the right thing.

- **Learn to send Qi downwards**. Meditating[3] is a start, but **deep slow breathing** does it too, as does learning to

3. http://www.acupuncture-points.org/meditation.html

concentrate on the sensations in your soles as you walk, in your palms as your hold things, in your finger-tips as you stroke things.

- **Balancing mind waves** – binaural waves[4].

- **Company** that is calming and supportive -eg Counselling.

- **Avoid moxa**[5]. Moxibustion is a great therapy in Chinese medicine, but unless you know exactly where to do it, (and if you are very Yin deficient there are not many places and some of them are on your back) don't do it. It is too Yang for you.

- **Avoid too much Heat** such as sauna, sunbathing for too long in the hot sun (even hot baths are inadvisable to start with although mild warmth does help to lower your blood pressure). Sunbathing is also important for everyone, but limit yourself to short periods to begin with and avoid it if it quickly over-heats you.

- **Exercise** that strengthens and steadies, such as:

- *Non-competitive*

- *Steady deep breathing*

- *Walking meditation[6]*

- *Keeps body flexible[7] so that Qi can flow and lead Blood, moving Blood around and thereby nourishing your Yin tissue; pilates.*

- *Resistance training or light weight-lifting – but only when you are ready!*

- *Qi Gong*

4. I use those provided by http://www.centerpointe.com
5. http://www.acupuncture-points.org/moxibustion.html
6. Useful at any time, but especially when travelling. I learned it at the Buddhist Society in London but any good meditation teacher will show you how. As with all forms of meditation, you need to practise it, ready for the emergency situation!
7. Yoga and Tai Chi, or read Appendix 10 in my book ' Qi Stagnation - Signs of Stress' for a quick spine rejuvenation exercise

- **Cool shower**[8]
- **Avoid exhaustion**, eg long-distance running
- **YANG!** = Doing something about it! (To increase Yin, increase Yang but be sure to take the correct – ie conducive – Yang action!) This means that you won't get better unless you do something about it! Some alteration in your behaviour or habits must happen or you will just get worse. Such a change is Yang. Use Yang to change and enhance Yin.

What about when Yin Deficiency leads to Empty Heat (explained above)?

For example, Empty Heat has a chronic tendency to dryness in the nose later becoming a chronic sore throat. What disease pictures fit this? Chapter 3 listed some of the conditions that may be recognised as being at least partially due to yin deficiency. Now that you have more familiarity with yin deficiency, the following are disease pictures recognised in Western medicine that may sooner or later carry aspects of *Yin deficiency with empty Heat*.

- Chronic disease in general, especially if it appears with inflammation or tissue destruction
- Many diseases of ageing, eczema, loss of hair and teeth, arterial calcification and erosion
- Mild inflammation accompanying many other conditions, including cancer
- ADHD
- Dementia
- Tendency for blood to coagulate

8. See http://www.acupuncture-points.org/cold-showers.html for more on why and how to take a cool/cold shower

- Osteo-arthritis and osteo-porosis

- Vaginitis, chronic

NB X-Ray treatment can burn tissues, reinforcing the tendency to Yin deficiency and empty heat.

What have we discovered that stimulates Yin?

Just as in the West huge investment has been made in rejuvenation (think of skin cream; botox and youth serums; blood from young mice injected into old mice to make them behave as if younger[9]; hormone replacement therapy and human growth hormone therapy; nutritional supplementation and nutriceuticals), so people grounded in Chinese medicine have spent substantial periods of their lives searching for how to prevent ageing and consumption of Yin!

We aren't doing anything new!

Apart from mental self-control, the ancients were really searching for ways to produce more Jing – Life Essence[10]. They worried less about just Yin deficiency. Life requires Yin and Yang and Jing Essence supplies both. So they mainly concentrated on Jing.

There are actions that strengthen, or seem to prolong Jing, and in so doing help Yin. Some are mentioned above, including Tai Qi and Qigong[11], proper nutrition, a steady attitude to life, meditation, and supportive, loving relationships.

They also developed herbs. However, although the following herbs, to a greater or lesser extent, strengthen Yin, each does other things too.

A herb that strengthens Yin will tend to slow things down, will moisturise and 'make heavy'. That heaviness makes Yang

9. http://med.stanford.edu/news/all-news/2014/05/infusion-of-young-blood-recharges-brains-of-old-mice-study-finds.html
10. http://www.acupuncture-points.org/jing-essence.html
11. However, the benefits from Tai Chi and Qigong take time to appear.

have to work harder to deal with it. So I doubt if experienced herbalists ever give Yin herbs on their own.

Anyone trained in Chinese herbalism would automatically use formulae that were balanced as between moisturising and drying, between heavy and light, between Yin and Yang. In particular, the formula would be adjusted to the individual needs of the patient.

Herbs by their nature are concentrated in action, otherwise we would use them as food. They often carry only limited nutrition, but they pack a punch. So they should be treated with respect.

One classic herbal formula in Chinese medicine is used as the basis for many treatments to strengthen Yin. It is always adjusted according to the diagnosed needs of the patient.

This is *Bu Wei di Huang tan* – 'Six Ingredients with Rehmannia' tea. This has the overall aim of nourishing Liver and Kidney Yin, especially the latter. Of the different herbs in the formula, however, *only one herb actually nourishes Yin*. The others all balance or stabilise this action or make the formula easier to digest. (See chapter 10 for a more detailed explanation of how this formula works.)

Why? Because as explained above, very Yin substances slow the body's Yang down. There is no point in so increasing Yin that, having done so, you can't move! Over the millennia Chinese herbalists acquired huge experience of how to deal with syndromes like Yin deficiency. I urge readers not to try to 'do it yourself'. Please consult someone experienced!

Acupuncturists also know which points work to strengthen Yin. Here again, balance is needed to maintain health. Treating a strongly Yin acupuncture point without also using other points to balance it earns few thanks because the patient feels exhausted, heavy, tired and a bit depressed.

What is clear is that nearly all such treatments derived from Chinese medicine aim, at least in part, to strengthen Blood.

Blood carries Qi within it, and both are needed to effect change. Compared to Qi, Blood is Yin. It is through the concept of Blood (capital 'B')[12] – though scientists don't think of blood (lower case 'b') the same way – that Western medicine is realising how to deal with ageing.

HRT – hormone replacement therapy – is a major step in this direction. Many women have blessed its effects. However, what I call the Primary and Secondary effect[13] of any medicine can bedevil women who take it. As we are discovering, the Secondary effects of HRT are many and varied, and some are dangerous.

To the extent HRT is Yin strengthening, it can increase other Yin actions in the body, for instance in the case of *oestrogen;* fluid retention; bloating; breast distension; indigestion (probably from lowered acid) and – towards the extreme – the formation of thrombo-embolisms (blood clots in the veins), with stroke, heart disease and cancerous tumours.

For *progesterone*, which appears to be slightly more Yang, there are also mood swings, depression and acne. Not surprisingly, amongst the advice given is advice to increase Yang activity, for instance to take exercise, to stretch, and to take HRT when eating meals, which dilutes its speed of delivery. (Exercise helps to move Qi and dissipate Heat, such as occur in many forms of depression and acne.)

Another piece of advice (bad advice in my opinion) is to eat a low-fat, high carbohydrate diet to reduce breast distension: that diet is likely to be high in foods that rapidly become sugar in the blood, supplying temporary Yang. (Fortunately, such a diet is increasingly discouraged because a secondary action of sugar is to increase weight.)

Our experience with HRT shows that concentrated medicines, herbs and even probably nutriceuticals should all be given only

12. http://www.acupuncture-points.org/blood.html
13. For more on this interesting topic, see http://www.acupuncture-points.org/primary-and-secondary-actions.html

with other herbs or foods to balance their action, or else be balanced in some other way, for example by exercise or with acupuncture points to counteract the intensity of the Yin action.

It is likely that every strongly Yin medicine or herb needs to be balanced, as explained, which is why the Chinese sought not a specific Yin medicine but a **Jing medicine**.

JING Medicine

The classical Chinese texts on the subject suggest that you need about 8 pints of good fresh blood to create one drop of Jing. They did not, (I think) mean this literally: just that Jing is hard to create. But the underlying point is that to get the Jing you have to make the Blood, which requires a range of actions[14].

Input to Blood comes not just from what we eat and drink, but from how healthy our body is, and how healthily our Energy organs – Stomach, Spleen, Kidney Fire, Lungs and Heart, all of which contribute – can make it.

So, for example, to improve Jing we need to keep our Lungs and Heart in order. We can do that with good breathing, right loving, meditation, right living, good exercise and food etc.

The inclusion in the list of Stomach and Spleen means that a good digestion is vital, and so are sensible, regular eating habits, and of course, what we put in our mouths must be high quality. Most people in search of the magic bullet to 'cure' Yin deficiency think solely of the food or herb or medicine in question, but all the others are as important.

This means that genetic research to improve and prolong the health of these Energy organs will probably be as or more effective than swallowing the right substance: or at least as fruitful a line of investigation as looking for the magic food or bullet! The problem is that genetic alteration is massively

14. These are described at http://www.acupuncture-points.org/blood.html

Yang in action with the potential for huge and unknown consequences, (like many Yang actions).

In the natural course of things, in nature, strongly Yang actions work out over Time and in Space. If we make genetic alterations we might not see their results for many generations. (However, we do have computers, which can hasten our prognostications.)

So injecting old mice with blood from young mice is not in itself a bad idea. I can foresee trouble, however, if we start producing babies to provide blood for their elders!

If we could make blood identical to the older person's blood but 'younger', that would solve this problem. However, that begs the question: how do you do it?

Of course, Yin deficiency is not the same as the problems that come with ageing, though it is often one of them. Ageing, in Chinese medicine, occurs as different syndromes occur or recur. One is Blood Stasis[15], another is Kidney deficiency[16], followed by Jing[17] deficiency. Blood syndromes are part of both Yin deficiency and ageing.

More Esoteric Practices

Listed above are various suggestions for strengthening Yin. However, the *priority is to balance Yin **and** Yang*. This is so that they can more easily support one another, stand up to one another, and in extremes, flow into or transform into one another.

Chinese literature is full of books and advice on this. Nowadays we live in an era of immediate gratification but despite thousands of years, nobody seems to have come up with a quick way either to strengthen Yin or to balance it with Yang. There are plenty of slow ways.

Some of these ways seem to give the impression of progress and several of them are forms of meditation. Unless under

15. http://www.acupuncture-points.org/blood-stasis.html
16. http://www.acupuncture-points.org/kidney-function.html
17. http://www.acupuncture-points.org/jing-essence.html

regular trusted guidance, the following are not recommended for those who are emotionally unbalanced or mentally ill:

- Vipassana meditation: this has become widely practised in the West as Mindulfness meditation.

- Walking meditation, already mentioned above. This involves a simple though powerful method of breathing meditation, being practised as one walks.

- Microcosmic meditation[18]. This is usually practised as part of a series of other practices aimed at fostering Qi, which can then be used to circulate under conscious control or, perhaps better put, under conscious awareness, from the abdomen downwards, then up the back, over and through the head, then down the front of the body, returning to the abdomen.

But even with these methods, *one must set aside a period of time regularly to practise.* Ancient advice suggests they should be done upright rather than lying. Results come slowly but can seem to come less slowly than with some other methods.

Because some very assiduous Chinese have been searching for thousands of years for a 'magic' food for Yin deficiency and/or Jing essence I don't hold great hope for nutrition on its own being able to answer our problem, but that's what the next chapter is about. At least they've found out what doesn't work.

18. Watch at https://youtu.be/nzoPhu-Kr-Q

Nutrition and Yin Deficiency

Good Eating Habits

Think back to when you were a baby! If your parents were conscientious, they would have provided you with a warm, loving environment and regular food, which you could eat at your own pace, and enough time to play, move around, explore, and then sleep. So treat yourself a bit like that!

- Regular habits! That means that most people should eat, for severe Yin deficiency, small amounts of food not too frequently. Even although your Yin energies are depleted, over-eating will exhaust you. Give yourself time to digest what you eat properly. Avoid snacking[1]. Both Stomach and Spleen Yang need Yin resources to do their work. As you are short of Yin which supplies Yang with the power to function, don't make Yang work too hard. Eat small quantities regularly rather than huge quantities occasionally, (but don't

---

1. Our ancestors lacked a source of food to eat 24/7. They survived feasts and famines. Your genes evolved to deal with this, not with constant feasting - ie food on tap at any time. Diabetes is much more likely nowadays with 24-hour snacking, especially if on refined carbohydrates. Also, small meals put less of a load on your Stomach Yang energy, which is the first of your energies to work on the food you swallow, and on Spleen Yang, which continues the process after that first stage, to make Blood[footnote] See http://www.acupuncture-points.org/blood.html

eat small snacks continuously through the day). Modern research shows that fasting between meals has merits for most people.

- Make sure the food is nutritious and properly prepared. Your genes, developed over millennia, have not yet adapted to the modern fast-food diet promoted by advertisers. Eat fresh whole foods, preferably organic and sustainably produced, and processed and refined as little as possible.

- If you are the cook, buy your food from reliable suppliers. Cook it without haste - make the preparation a time for reflection and enjoying yourself[2].

- Food ready for preparation and cooking should be as natural as possible.

- Eat food that, when acquired, is fresh and looks like it was immediately after being picked or killed. Use fresh vegetables, fruit and meat as far as possible.

- Try to avoid food that contains artificial additives such as colouring, preservatives, added flavours, herbicides, pesticides and fertilisers. Unfortunately, these are almost impossible to avoid unless you eat organic food, which may not be an option for you. But non-organic food can be more nutritious than organic food if the latter comes from earth that has not yet regained its original patency. The problem is that fertilisers are not always well balanced: the basic three main minerals (potassium, nitrogen and phosphorus) boost growth but don't contain other vital minerals that plants depend on and which make them healthy and consequently nutritious for you. For example, selenium deficiency was discovered to be a cause of cancer in China in an area where the earth was deficient in the mineral[3].

2. Processing of food developed mainly in the 20th century as a way of prolonging shelf-life. Partly this worked because vermin didn't like it. If rats won't eat it, should you?
3. https://link.springer.com/article/10.1007/BF02916544#page-1

- Sweeteners: if artificial, avoid them. If natural, take in very small quantities, or not at all. Natural sweeteners give you a very temporary boost but soon burn you out. Artificial sweeteners such as aspartame may lack calories and may make food more palatable but they cause many illnesses – see 'Sweet Misery – A Poisoned World' DVD[4]. Aspartane affects protein synthesis and its by-products cross the blood-brain barrier and may confuse thinking, to say the least.

- Sugars from corn and honey: although these are from natural sources, they are still sugars. Sugars like this are quick but empty energy. If your body cannot use them through physical exertion, it tends to turn them to fat, with the prospect of diabetes. In time it reduces your Spleen's viability.

- Salt and pepper - common condiments on your table. You need salt, but not much as most natural foods contain quantities absorbed naturally from the earth. Pepper can supply warmth ie Yang to a dish, helping your Stomach Yang. But it is easy to become dependent on it, or on other warming spices, so do not take too much.

- Chemicals that encourage you to eat more? So-called 'Organic' food is preferable for a variety of reasons. It comes from soil that has not been depleted by intensive farming using fertilisers, pesticides, herbicides etc. The earth contains fungus spores and tendrils (Mycorrhizae) that work with a plant's roots to bring to the plant more nutrients from the soil than its roots can normally reach, and in return the plant supplies the fungus with carbohydrates and other growth factors. Together they keep the soil healthy for plants, insects, worms and animals: including you and me. (Of course, one of the best natural fertilisers in the past came from human and animal faeces, and gardens fertilised

4. https://www.youtube.com/watch?v=toKyRlpmG7A

this way were often noticeably more productive than modern gardens, with plants that grew bigger and more healthily.) Use of artificial fertilisers, pesticides, herbicides etc kills off the mycorrhizae: that means the farmer has to increase the quantity of fertilisers he uses, and then also use herbicides and pesticides to prevent the plants from dying, when in the past, organic farming produced more plants that were healthy, although they may not have looked as smart as we are now used to. Indeed, if a plant or fruit looks perfect, it has probably received a lot of loving non-organic attention that may be detrimental to your health. Fruit and plants that looks less than perfect, if grown naturally, are likely to be just as healthy, if not more so, than 'perfect' foods, because they have had to fight for existence, so contain a wide range of enzymes that repel attackers. Many of those enzymes are what make the plant really nutritious for us.

- Avoid huge meals. They put your system under a load it can do without. As you may have noticed, after a large meal you often feel sleepy. Partly that is due to your body pumping insulin into your blood to help absorb all the sugars you've eaten. That gives you a 'hypo'. But it also happens because your body is using so much energy to digest the food. That energy comes from your Yin supplies, just as what makes your car go fast comes from its fuel tank. Driving uphill fast in low gears makes the fuel gauge go down more quickly.

Avoidance of Yin draining foods, herbs and drugs

Yin draining substances are those that make you use your energy faster or more intensively, and prevent you from getting sufficient sleep and good rest. They include:

- Coffee[5] and caffeine, often added to drinks and medicines to keep you alert and 'buzzing': disastrous if you are Yin deficient! I strongly advise you to stop coffee altogether if you are Yin deficient. People who are Yin deficient and take coffee find they get very energetic for some hours then feel exhausted! Also, they often get noises in their ears, and sleep patterns are upset for several days each time after they have coffee.

- Other foods and drinks containing caffeine like substances, including tea. Even decaffeinated coffee and tea often still contain other stimulants. The later in the day that you take them, the more likely they are to prevent deep sleep. However, Chinese experience and observation of the effects of tea show that not all teas are equal. Some mild stimulation from good green tea, not stewed, appears less stimulating and may improve digestion. Similarly Mate Tea. However, these do still contain stimulants and someone who is *very* Yin deficient should avoid them.

- Spicy food can stimulate your body too much: spices are naturally warming. Taken in excess, spices can cause sweating which depletes Yin fluids. Even if they don't do that, they may warm you up too much to rest deeply. So avoid spicy food later in the day, or if you know you are sensitive to it. (How do you know that? Usually because it gives you loose, often smelly, stools later on or the next day.)

- Chinese ginseng is a great herb, used for millennia. Unfortunately, for many people it stimulates Yang too much, so avoid it until your Yin deficiency has gone. As you improve, if you are taking herbs from an experienced Chinese herbalist, you may find that he or she starts using Ginseng in formulae for you – but very seldom on its own. Also, good ginseng is expensive.

- Social drugs that put you on a 'high'.

5. http://www.acupuncture-points.org/coffee.html

- Greasy and oily foods. These produce Heat, Damp and Phlegm which in Chinese medicine are said to injure the Spleen and Stomach energies. Without healthy Spleen and Stomach energies you cannot digest food. However, you do most definitely need fats in you diet, see below.

- Alcohol: better avoided, although in small quantities it does often ease Qi Stagnation[6] which, for many, contributes to Yin deficiency. Many people find that alcohol before bedtime helps them to go to sleep. This may be true, but it is usually too 'heating' in Chinese medicine, so prevents proper, deep, restful, recuperating sleep.

- Medications that interfere with your body's ability to achieve proper rest or nutrition. Many prescribed medications interfere with sleep patterns, causing restless sleep, or making you too hot, or making you sweat without cause. Sweating when you aren't hot, or when you don't have a cold, wastes precious energy, especially Yin-type energy, which you certainly don't need to lose!

- Many prescribed medications interfere also with how well your body absorbs food. Some make you less hungry – so you don't eat what you need; others either kill off good bacteria in your gut that you do need; or make food pass through you too fast for your bowels to absorb what they need; or make you constipated so that you cannot get rid of debris; or upset the acid/alkali and enzyme balances considered essential for proper digestion.

Eat warm food or cooked and eaten warm

To be nutritious, food must be absorbable.

When you are Yin deficient, although you may not have a

6. For much more on this important topic for Yin-deficient people, see http://www.acupuncture-points.org/qi-stagnation.html or my book on it, 'Qi Stagnation - Signs of Stress', appendix 4.

definable illness in terms of Western medicine, you are still ill, from a Chinese medicine point of view. Cold, icy food and raw food are considered harder to digest than cooked, warm food. (Of course, when you are perfectly well, cold, raw food may not be a problem, and on a hot day in summer, can be eaten by even someone who is yin deficient – if it is well-chewed and in small quantities.)

To digest food, your body needs ample supplies of Yang energy, specifically Stomach Yang, and very cold food absorbs all this Yang. Your body has to make more of it, and guess where it comes from? Right! Your supplies of Yin! So cook your food and eat it warm.

Eat when quiet and relaxed

Nowadays we fit food around our work. In ideal times in the past, eating was an event, a time with family/friends to be relished, a time to talk and swap ideas, to laugh and relax. Then, after a rest, you started work again.

We seem to have lost that. We eat merely to fuel ourselves, omitting the important social and time benefits. In Chinese medicine theory there is a strong suggestion, that the social dimension comes before the food and digestion, that it has priority and that a strong social side actually benefits digestion.

In Chinese medicine this theory - Five Element theory, which is probably as old as Yin/Yang theory - makes Fire the 'mother' of Earth. Fire symbolises many things, including social intercourse. It comes before Earth, signifying digestion and nourishment.

The same theory suggests that after eating, we need space/ time before getting back to work. So after eating, take a walk for 15 minutes, or have a short nap: but preferably take the walk, because the air you breathe supplies oxygen which your body needs for good digestion. [Five Element theory also makes

Earth the Mother of Metal which includes the actions of the Lungs and the Large Intestine and emphasises the need for Air and Space. So after food, give yourself space and benefit from inhaled, fresh air.].

This means it is better NOT to

- Eat while working
- Eat in a rush
- Eat fast foods
- Eat when tired
- Eat when arguing
- Eat when upset
- Eat while exercising

So what SHOULD you eat?

For your body to replace the missing Yin, it needs food that is very nutritious, cooked and prepared properly, then chewed and eaten regularly, and digested fully. It needs a healthy digestion and good food.

Bear in mind that, even with exactly the right foods, your body will take time to repair itself. Digesting and absorbing food is a Yin-type process so is hard to hurry. (Not to be confused with the quick, but ultimately exhausting boost that stimulants provide. You most definitely should not take stimulants! See earlier in this chapter.)

Your body needs foods that provide balanced nutrition. Of course, in Western food science this means that protein, carbohydrate, vitamin, mineral, and fat are available in the right proportions.

When should you eat?

Some of what follows repeats what has gone before, from a slightly different perspective.
Do not eat when:

- Tired. If tired, take a small snack and rest for a while, then eat a larger meal. A small snack might be a little soup (Miso soup has great qualities, like Chicken soup) or a few oat biscuits, or a little brown rice, previously well-prepared, or the Chinese form of rice porridge.

- Inebriated by alcohol (Mind you, if you're intoxicated, you may not be in a condition to decide what is good and what is not!)

- Intoxicated with drugs

If you are tired and 'deficient', do not eat too much at a time. Eating a large meal, especially before sleeping is counter-productive because it may cause Food Retention[7], which leads to waking often and un-refreshing sleep.

A small meal before sleep may help Yin- and Blood-deficient people. Some almonds, or almond milk (taken warm); a milky drink perhaps; or try some olive oil, perhaps on rye bread with fresh tomato, all chewed well. In Chinese medicine, there is a traditional suggestion that the largest meals be taken in the morning, but with very Yin-deficient conditions, this is less important.

The Energy of Food

In Chinese medicine, besides the nutritional value of food, there is an important additional dimension - *that foods of balanced energies should be eaten*.

7. See http://www.acupuncture-points.org/food-retention.html

Good nutrition, in Chinese medicine, and specifically for mending a deficiency, recognises individual differences and implies the need for a balance between the different kinds of food energy. Chinese medicine stresses the total regime, including nutrition, and not miracle cures.

Some Theory!

Now comes a bit of theory. You don't have to master it, although if you do, it may make it easier to decide which foods you need.

As regards Yin deficiency, food energies in Chinese medicine are described in various ways:

- Yin and Yang foods ie cooling or warming

- Taste: 6 flavours, each of which also favours Yin or Yang

- Moist or dry

The six flavours (one, not shown in the table 1, being neutral) each affect one of the channels and energy organs.

Chapter 9 Table 1

Chapter 9, Table 1	Channel/ Energy Organ	Function	Examples of Use
Bitter	Heart and Small Intestine	Dries Damp, clear Heat; stimulates appetite; strengthens the Lungs, induces diarrhoea; sedates	Hot or Damp diseases including hot, dry constipation and Qi stagnation.
Sweet	Spleen and Stomach	Tonifying, harmonises and slows; moisturises and nourishes	Mildly benefits deficiency conditions; muscle pain and spasm
Pungent	Lungs and Large Intestine	Dispersing and moving, up and out; assists circulation; stimulates appetite	Externally caused diseases like colds and from bacteria or viruses

		Descends and flows energy	
Salty	Kidney and Bladder	Descends and flows energy downward; dissipates hardness and accumulation; promotes bowel movements	TB; constipation
Sour	Liver and Gallbladder	Contracts and astringes; controls discharges including sweating and nasal fluids	Empty conditions; deficiency

- Do not misunderstand Table 1 above! The words on the left (pungent, sweet, salty, sour, bitter) might make you think that by eating daily one small cardamom (Pungent), a few grains each of sugar (Sweet), a pinch of salt (Salty), some grains of instant coffee (Bitter) and a drop of lemon juice (Sour) you could be eating a balanced diet with nothing but good health to look forward to! However, those examples are extreme forms of each taste.

- When considering a food's energy, the Chinese considered a whole range of issues, including the *acupuncture channel* that the food 'entered into', *how dry or moisturising* it was, *in which direction* (up, down, inwards or outwards) a food worked and a whole lot more[8]. One of the extra considerations was *which Energy Organs*[9] a food 'entered' and hence what its nature was. The five tastes 'are' the five natures. From the above you might think that eating salt would ease constipation but that, emphatically, is not what is meant. However, if you eat rather more foods considered in Chinese medicine to possess the Salty *taste*, such as seaweed, pork, abalone and barley, you will gradually heal your intestines and in due course, with a good diet, your bowel motions will normalise. The other ingredients in your good diet would include representatives from all the flavours, not just the Salty flavour, and all the foods eaten would be in their original raw, organically-grown, state when

8. If you can accept that deep breathing calms you, in other words it sends energy downwards, then, for the sake of argument, please accept that foods can also direct energies up or down, though more gently!

9. http://www.acupuncture-points.org/zang-fu.html

prepared and cooked (... with no additives, flavourings, preservatives ...).

How a flavour works depends on which energy is applied:

- Cold energy (eg freezing or chilling a food) forms cold and cools internal organs, clears heat and sedates Fire. Detoxifying.
- Cool energy (eg cool room temperature) reduces Heat more gently than Cold food.
- Warm energy (eg heating or cooking food) disperses Cold and restores Yang energy.
- Hot energy (eg roasting, adding hot spices): creates heat and warms.

For example a food can have the same energy but a different effect:

- Warm and Sweet food tonifies Qi
- Cold and Sweet food cools Heat
- Some foods have different flavours but the same energy
- Bitter and Cold food cools Heat
- Pungent and Cold food sedates Heat and Wind

Chapter 9, Table 2

Flavour	Energy Generated	Action in the Body	Disease Conditions
Pungent and Sweet	Warm, Hot	Removes Cold and promotes Yang	Yin Excess and Yang deficient
Sweet, Salty	**Cold**	**Nourishes Yin**	**Yin Deficient**
Sour, Bitter	Cold	Clears Heat	Yang Excess
Sweet	Warm	Assists Qi	Qi Deficiency

Sweet and Cold	Cold	Reduces Heat	Blood Deficiency
Sour	Warm	Moves Blood	Blood stagnation eg clotting

(Just for interest, notice that the pungent flavour helps to clear Yin excess. Hence, some Chinese doctors recommended that their patients who had quantities of cold phlegm in their chests should smoke tobacco - cigarettes - to warm and disperse the fluids there (yin excess). This was **not** a long-term recommendation to smoke but a medical intervention of the help-yourself variety, *short-term*: very pragmatic is Chinese medicine!)

From the table above (Table 2) one can see that for Yin and Blood deficiencies, which are closely related, foods that are by and large classified as sweet, slightly salty and cold are beneficial.

That does not mean they should be taken cold! Eat them cooked and warm! Remember that too much Cold food destroys Yang energy. If you are Yin deficient you will have *comparatively* more Yang than Yin, but even so, you are probably deficient in both.

You can often remove the damaging effects of Coldness from a food by combining it with a warming herb like Ginger, which is what herbal formulae prepared the Chinese way aim to do. You might think that Ginger here would be too warming, thereby wasting the Cold energy of the food you are eating.

So it would, if taken in great quantity or in the form of dried, powdered, ginger. But if you are adding just a thin slice of ginger root, chopped small, during cooking, it won't overwhelm the Yin quality and will be enough to assist your Stomach and Spleen Yang to digest it.

To take an example. Tea (whether Indian or Chinese) is said to have a Cool energy. Even when drunk warm or hot, straight from the kettle/pot, it has a Cooling energy. For one thing it makes you urinate, for another, it can make you perspire, both of which are cooling in their action.

In fact, the hotter you take it the more likely it will be to make you perspire. However, don't get confused by the temperature at which you take it, because some warming foods, like strong spices from Asia and Central America, can also make you perspire: food and herbal medicine takes knowledge and experience to practise.

For Yin deficiency purposes, just try to eat the appropriate foods warm to the touch and occasionally add ginger root in small quantities to assist your digestion, especially if the food is classified as Cold in its nature. So assist your Yang energy by eating food cooked and warm.

(By the way, the sixth, neutral, flavour is also called 'mild' and it encourages the other flavours to be desired and easily digested. For the purposes of this book you can ignore it.)

The five main flavours can be split into two groups, Yin and Yang:

Chapter 9 Table 3

Chapter 9 Table 3	Flavour	Function
Yang	Mild	Moves fluids, so increases urination
Yang	Sweet, pungent	Disperses, mainly by encouraging perspiration
Yin	Salty, bitter, sour	Descends energy, so can produce diarrhoea

The theory suggests that if a disease is Yang, in other words, Hot, one should use Yin foods to balance it - and reduce the amount of Yang foods.

Conversely, in excess Yin diseases, where there is too much Yin (eg oedema,) Yang foods should be taken, as these make you urinate it out: also, reduce foods that are strongly Yin in nature. (So, for the patients with cold fluids in their chests mentioned above, who were recommended to smoke tobacco, they most *definitely* would have been advised against eating ice-cream!)

Yang foods tend to push energy upwards and outwards (eg perspiration) whereas too many Yin foods send it down (eg diarrhoea). This explains why, if you are Yin deficient and eat too many Yin-type foods, without also taking some Yang type foods, the Yin-type foods will pass straight through you, or at least will do little to improve your Yin-deficient status.

What about the strength of the taste and smell and the temperature of the food?

Chapter 9, Table 4

Chapter 9, Table 4	Smell and Taste	Temperature
Yin-type foods	Mild	Cold
Yang-type foods	Strong	Hot

Table 4 describes the nature of the foods themselves, not what alterations in their actions happen when you prepare and cook them in different ways, such as stir-frying a Yin-type food, which will reduce the intensity of its Yin nature by applying some Yang - Heating qualities to it.

The above is only a brief introduction to the energetic action of foods. Some of it is a bit technical and may repay re-reading.

In Appendix 1 is a list of foods that, in general, are classified in Chinese medicine as being Sweet and Salty and Cold: on the whole their movement is downwards and inwards, helping to tonify Yin. The list also includes some foods that are warming and hot, for information and because they are also needed to balance the effects of too much Yin-tonifying food.

From the above, you will realise that taken in excess, or eaten too cold, foods with Sweet, Salty and Cold natures can produce downward movement more powerful than their inward movement, leading to diarrhoea; also they may make you feel cold and more susceptible to cold diseases.

In addition, Yin-tonifying foods deplete Yang, which leads to food stagnation. You need to balance Yin-tonifying foods with some Yang-tonifying foods.

I have also included some foods that, even though their main function may be warming, also tonify Blood. Without Blood support any Yin deficiency improvement will not last long.

If a food you want to know about is not listed, it means that no consensus on its action has yet been reached - or perhaps I forgot it. The list also excludes flavourings and other chemicals that did not exist in the past.

Oils and fats

I have not included much about oils and fats. These are excellent foods for Yin deficient people, but they should be either saturated fats as from many animal and vegetable sources, or unsaturated fats as from oily fish and many seeds. However, the more we know about foods the easier it is to be led astray.

In the past, people aimed to eat a wide range of foods naturally produced in nature. Nowadays most of us seldom if ever see our food being grown or raised.

We have become dependent for information on scientists and the government, well-meaning but influenced by large manufacturing marketing forces and the latest research.

In relation to oils and fats, although we should avoid trans-fats and hydrogenated fats, we should eat a wide range. However, in terms of unsaturated fats we should not eat too many Omega 6 fats over Omega 3 fats. The ideal ratio of Omega 3 to Omega 6 fats has not been decided, but probably should be 1:1 or 3:5 instead of what many eat, which is in the area of 1:10 or more. Ideally these fats should not be processed.

Stir-Frying?

It is only partially true that stir-frying destroys good fats and introduces bad fats. This occurs but not in any quantity. Stir-frying is a quick and convenient way of cooking that makes food more digestible. Arguably the minute amount of 'bad' fats[10] it creates does no harm and may do good!.

Nuts are good! Though many are slightly heating, they contain huge amounts of beneficial nutrients, including oils. Taken with other more cooling foods they provide a range of benefits that are hard to match.

The list contains many foods common in Chinese food-stores but with which Westerners are unfamiliar. I suggest you admit ignorance and ask for help. Most first or second generation Chinese know how to prepare the Chinese foods, even if they have been lured away from their roots by the temptations of Western-style fast-food!

As a general rule:

- Yang enhancing foods tend to grow above ground, in the rain and sun: for example, grains, nuts, seeds and fruits.

- Green vegetables are mostly grown at ground level so are less Yang usually.

- Yin enhancing plants grow underground, in the dark: tubers, roots.

- Yin enhancing foods tend to be wet and soft when raw.

- Yang enhancing foods tend to by spicy, dry and hard.

Even with this general rule, you may be surprised at some of the actions. Cardamon, for example, is considered to be Yin in nature, but warming. Of course, being a herb it provides little of nutritional value but lots of energetic value, so use it with more

10. See 'Cooking and Transfats' on letters page of Scientific American July 2014.

nutritious Yin-type foods to warm them and leaven their action for you.

As you will be gathering, the energetics of food can be subtle and require skill and time. *(Skill and Time - Yin words.)*

So even with food, for Yin deficiency there is really no quick fix.

CHAPTER 10

Help for Yin Deficiency

Your aim is to find a way to help you to slow down, to calm and steady your system and, eventually, to strengthen it so that it becomes less Yin deficient and you become more resilient. However, a word of warning! I urge you to take advice. Someone else may have a more objective perspective than you. Bear in mind that "sick people take sick decisions".

You may not be sick in the ordinary sense of the word, but if you are Yin deficient you are out of balance, which in Chinese medicine is the first stage of becoming 'sick'.

I also urge you **not** to try to advance on too many fronts at once. For example, do not take homoeopathic remedies while also receiving acupuncture or herbs. They work in ways that are so close that they may clash, or your therapist may not know from which actions results are flowing, causing confusion and prolonging the time you take to get better.

1/ **Stress**: stress tightens you up; it causes Qi to stagnate; stagnant Qi emerges as what in Chinese medicine are called symptoms of 'Wind' or 'Heat'[1]. Both of these forms are Yang-type energies, which test your Yin resources. If your body or self-management won't let Stagnant Qi escape by

---

1. For more on these see http://www.acupuncture-points.org/wind.html and
http://www.acupuncture-points.org/Heat.html

healthy means, it implodes, leading to disease that is more deep-seated and harder to cure. This more chronic form of disease drains your resources, leading eventually to Jing Essence[2] deficiency, including Yin deficiency. The excess Yang caused by Stagnant Qi is also a drain on any existing Yin deficiency. My book 'Qi Stagnation – Signs of Stress' explains much more about Stress and how your stagnant – trapped – energy can be harnessed for good and can even lead to transformation in your outlook and life.

2/ **Acupuncture**[3] has been used for thousands of years. Used as understood by Traditional Chinese medicine, (and similar forms of acupuncture such as have developed in Japan, Vietnam and Korea) it aims to balance Yin and Yang forces in your body. Although often not yet accepted by Western medical doctors, it allows acupuncturists to contact and stabilise what they conceive of as an invisible web of channels of energy that manages the body. There are many acupuncture points for this. Some are powerful points that, in effect, calm Yang, others help Yin to mend faster, others help clear Empty Heat. Still others, just as powerful in their own ways, adjust the way you and your body work so that you take the appropriate decisions to mend your ways and adjust to a steadier and more Yin-enhancing lifestyle. Of course, when a diagnosis has been reached it may cover many other conditions from which you are suffering and help you to recover from them too.

3/ **NLP Neurolinguistic Programming** and somewhat similar forms of psychological help such as Cognitive Behavioural Therapy (CBT) can teach you how to behave and think differently[4]. They both require professional help. Learning to behave differently can take time but these therapies can be enormously helpful. They help you re-programme yourself.

---

2. http://www.acupuncture-points.org/jing-essence.html
3. http://www.acupuncture-points.org/what-is-acupuncture.html
4. . The Chinese used to call Counselling 're-education'!

4/ **Herbs**[5] have been used for thousands of years and their qualities are well understood.

Modern herbs are now mass-produced for a huge worldwide market and, because producing them has lead to industrial processes of farming, it is possible that many herbs lack the quality that they once had when harvested in the wild. Furthermore, herbs cultivated intensively can suffer from the same problems as food so cultivated, including from the use of herbicides, pesticides, artificial fertilisers, and fungicides etc.

Still, Chinese medicine has many herbs that assist your body to improve its Yin energy but they are never, or very seldom, given on their own. Any competent herbalist using Chinese medicine theories would adjust herbal formulae according to the particular diagnosis for a given patient. Such famous 'starting-place' formulae include *si wu tang* that nourishes the Blood and *liu wei di huang wan* that nourishes and tonifies Yin. Chinese medicine is subtle and powerful and I strongly recommend that you do not self-medicate: doing so can be expensive and unproductive.

To explain more about how Chinese herbs work, consider *liu wei di huang wan*. This is a tonic specifically for Kidney and Liver Yin deficiency, (so if your Yin deficiency is not much of this kind it may not help.) The classical recipe contains six herbs, each of which has a very definite reason for being in the formula and in the right proportions. Some herbs are considered to support the main function, others balance it or make it more digestible. You would never take the main herb in this formula on its own because it is too strongly Yin and indigestible. The formulae is in two parts, each of three herbs.

First group of herbs in the formula:

- *Shu di huang (Radix Rehmanniae Glutinosae Conquitae)* is in the recipe because it so strongly supports Jing and Kidney

5. http://www.acupuncture-points.org/chinese-herbs.html

Yin. However it is very indigestible so other herbs in the formula balance this.

- *Shan zhu yu (Fructus Cornii Officinalis)* is in the formula because it tends to prevent loss of Jing by an importunate Liver energy[6], so enabling Yin to build up in the Kidneys. This herb is, however, a rather warming type of herb so *mu dan pi* from the second half of the formula helps to balance this by cooling.

- *Shan yao (Radix Dioscoreae Oppositae)* the third herb in the first group, benefits the Spleen. The Spleen[7] energy in Chinese medicine has many important duties, but one of them is to keep things in place. In this case it helps the Spleen to bind or stabilise the Jing. Incidentally it also moistens the Lung (helps Lung Yin[8]) and 'firms' the Kidneys[9].

The second group of herbs making up this formula has a slightly different purpose. Given that the first group helps to hold things in place, the second group makes sure that not too much is held in place. It ensures that, for all there is a build-up of Yin, any sign, for example of oedema (an excess of Yin), is quickly resolved.

- *Fu ling (Sclerotium Poriae Cocos)*, one of the most widely used herbs in Chinese medicine, is included to prevent any build-up of Damp[10] (another form of excess Yin). It is also known to work well with Shan Yao, from the first half of the formula. Fu Ling has other qualities, one of which is to calm the mind, always useful if there is Yin deficiency.

- *Mu dan pi (Cortex Moutan Radicis)* is particularly good at clearing any signs of excess Yang in the form of Liver

6. See also http://www.acupuncture-points.org/liver-functions.html
7. http://www.acupuncture-points.org/spleen.html
8. http://www.acupuncture-points.org/lung-yin.html
9. http://www.acupuncture-points.org/kidney-function.html
10. http://www.acupuncturepoints.org/damp.html

Fire[11] but it also works in tandem with *shan zhu yu* to prevent any sign of excess warmth which the latter herb without this regulator might otherwise build up.

- *Ze xie (Rhizoma Alismatis Orientalis)* does something similar to *mu dan pi* but in relation to Kidney Fire. It stops the very rich, heavy, cloying effects of *shu di huang* from clogging up the Kidney energy. Without this herb, the build up of Yin in the Kidneys might turn to Yang and consequently generate more heat, the last thing you want if you are Yin deficient! This herb also works well with *shan yao* to keep fluids moving, not allowing them to build up and lead to a local form of Yin excess – such as oedema – before the body has had time to strengthen its Yin qualities in general.

All the herbs in both groups have other qualities that benefit the general strategy behind the formula – I have only mentioned some of them. The first group are usually given in higher quantities than the second group but a herbalist using the formula would adjust it as he saw fit, according to the particular needs of the patient. He might add other herbs, or take out herbs, or replace some of them. Sometimes a formula is so adjusted that possibly only one or two of the original herbs remain from the classical formula!

Some Western herbs[12] can of course treat Yin deficiency. However, possibly because of the way Western herbs are prepared (often merely steeped in alcohol or water) compared with the Chinese equivalents, which are generally boiled, the Yin enhancing qualities of the Chinese herbs may be greater: perhaps boiling extracts more of the Yin-enhancing qualities.

However, against that, Western herbs are often kept in alcohol or water for considerable periods of time, which helps

11. http://www.acupuncture-points.org/liver-fire.html
12. For a fuller discussion of Western Herbs from the Chinese energetic perspective, read "The Energetics of Western Herbs" by Peter Holmes, Artemis Press.

to extract useful qualities and preserve enzymes and even vitamins that would be destroyed by boiling. Western herbalists are only slowly moving towards understanding which of their herbs enhance Jing, but some are known to assist Yin.

Herbs such as Hawthorn, Marjoram and Mistletoe are in many ways Yin tonics in that they work by stimulating the parasympathetic system. Mostly, these kinds of herbs are cooling, firming and steadying. They may not be specific enough for a given condition, for instance if a condition is typified by dryness (which might be Lung Yin deficiency) or by Empty Heat. So additional herbs, depending on the situation, would be added to provide moisture, possibly with other herbs that circulate Qi and/or with herbs that, for Empty Heat situations clear Heat and fever; also herbs to calm the spirit.

Doing it this way uses the experience of Chinese medicine for herbs outside the Chinese herbal tradition. At the same time as taking such a Yin tonic it would be sensible to avoid or reduce herbs that inhibit Yin, such as Angelica, Cypress, Hyssop, Lavender, Roman camomile and Thyme. These herbs contain powerful essential oils that are pungent and warm.

Beware Toxic Heavy Metals in herbs

Beware toxic heavy metals, not to say the remains of herbicides, pesticides and fungicides, present in some Chinese herbal over the counter products (and possibly in the raw herbs and formulae in countries where there are poor import restrictions.) Although there is increasing awareness of this, with governmental intervention and control in many countries, taking pills or products that contain no proper translation into your own language, eg English, puts you at a considerable disadvantage. In the UK nowadays, reputable Chinese herb importers guarantee that their herbs are free of heavy metals.

Herb Dosage vs Time

Shops that sell yin-enhancing herbs may benefit by selling

you more than you perhaps need. Remember that increasing your Yin energy takes time. Taking high doses of supposedly Yin-enhancing recipes may not increase the speed with which you improve and, in some cases, could slow it down, because, as explained, you need Yang energy herbs to help you absorb and utilise Yin-enhancing herbs.

American Ginseng *Panax quinquefolium*. This is known as American Ginseng although the herb bears no relation to Chinese Ginseng. However, it has both Yin and Yang enhancing qualities and if a single herb could be chosen for benefiting Yin, this might be it. However, people react to it in different ways because we all have different constitutions and what suits me might not suit you. Also, as demand increases, quality and results may deteriorate. As usual in Chinese medicine, it may work better if you take it in a formula designed specifically for you rather than if taken on its own.

5/ **Ancient disciplines** eg Yoga, Tai Qi, Qi Gong, Meditation

Over several thousand years, a number of traditions have emerged to help keep us fit (ie with Yin and Yang in balance) and to keep us calm and centred. While Yoga developed in India and Sri Lanka (and there are many kinds of Yoga, only one of which, Hatha, is predominantly physical), and while meditation has been taught in different ways in different cultures for untold centuries, in China the result was Qi gong and various forms of Tai Chi, both of which were informed by their grasp of the fundamental importance of the web of acupuncture channels for health.

a/ These traditional methods need time to learn and practise and require perseverance. Although their Yang-pacifying benefits can work fast, their Yin-enhancing benefits do not develop immediately. Only as your body and mind become stronger through diligent practice does your Yin grow tougher. At the same time, your Yin and Yang move into balance.

b/ Whether Tai Chi or Qi Gong arose first, the latter is

generally reckoned now to be the greater system, encompassing Tai Chi. Practising either over time and, for best results, under tuition, leads to lasting changes for the better.

c/ There is a modern tendency to combine many of these old systems with modern or scientifically-based regimes, making them faster to practise and with more emphasis on developing physical strength or grace. This change of emphasis works fine but because the end desired is different, the Yin enhancing benefits may be reduced or take longer to be achieved. Examples include Pilates and Gyrotonics.

d/ Learning to meditate[13] and learning to pray are not the same thing but have many similar benefits, the enhancement of a Yin-steadying mindset being one of them.

6/ Modern ways to increase Yin include **supplements**. In Chinese medicine part of the aim of herbal treatment is to nourish the Blood. The Blood then nourishes the Yin. So a good digestion and appropriate foods, (see chapter 9 and appendix 1), are important. If you have a poor digestion, improving your Yin/Yang balance will be much harder.

Many modern drugs suppress the symptoms of poor digestion without necessarily curing it, meaning that you have to continue the medication indefinitely. I suggest you try some of the alternative systems of medicine mentioned here. They may be able to reduce your dependence on medication if not cure you. Along the way they may open your eyes to a whole new way of thinking about life and health. Still, if medication is effective, and you cannot find an alternative, stick with it!

Nutritional supplements may be helpful, though good food is better, because our genes are adapted to food, and there is no question that supplements and nutriceuticals can be abused. Also, because they are concentrated forms of food, to some extent they can act like weak medication. As such there will be a Primary and a Secondary effect though this may not

13. See http://www.acupuncture-points.org/meditation.html

be noticeable for some time. The more balanced or food-like the supplement is, the less of a danger posed by the Primary and Secondary effects.

In general I prefer supplements that are as close to food as possible, and are preferably made from organic or chemical-free foods harvested at maturity and then concentrated by the removal of fibre and water so that the nutrients remain in the same proportions as in the original food. Such foods will be easier to digest and will yield their benefits more easily than concentrated vitamins and minerals taken individually, especially those manufactured. Your body probably absorbs more vitamin C from an apple than from a spoonful of vitamin C powder, because the apple contains thousands of other nutrients working together to help you absorb the vitamin, even though on the face of it, the apple contains a smaller amount of the vitamin.

However, if such supplements are too expensive or not available in your country, look for supplements that deal first with nerves, then with bones and proper brain function, and only then with supplements for muscle. Muscle – flesh – will then build on healthy bone and nerve. Muscles are not the first thing to concentrate on when strengthening Yin resilience, although later they are not unimportant, see 9 below.

Do not forget fluids, including oils and fats. Also water, but if your Yin is very deficient, probably so also is your Yang, and large amounts of water could put a strain on the latter. Get into the habit of, in effect, chewing the water you drink by which I mean you should take it a half-mouthful at a time and then swill it round your mouth as if it were food for a few seconds, properly mixing it with saliva and warming it before swallowing it. You will probably find that you need less water this way and your body will absorb it better. Also, the very act of 'chewing' the water slows you down!

7/ **Exercise** When you have put digestion and diet right, and your body is beginning to improve its most Yin resources such as marrow, brain and nerve, only then think about Exercise.

From an extreme Yin deficiency state, the first exercise you do is to walk! Walking makes your legs carry your weight, so encourages them to build bone and muscles to support it. Your thigh bones in particular have strong marrow-producing cells. Marrow is a very Yin resource and more of it assists your body to reduce its Yin deficiency.

Eventually, as bones and nerves improve your body will be able to support more flesh. Although you need fat to survive, you don't need obesity. How easily you tone or build muscle, and not extraneous fat, depends on your metabolism and lifestyle. You should, if Yin deficient, avoid activities that exhaust you. Instead take exercise that moves and stretches your joints and muscles, whilst keeping you calm and centred.

That is why Tai Chi is so good. Tai Chi is harder work than you may think, but not exhausting, and it tests just about every fibre in your body without strain. You can learn it from videos online, but far better from an experienced teacher/ practitioner. Regular, daily practice is important, just like good food.

An alternative is Hatha yoga but I regard Tai Chi as probably superior for Yin deficiency, because Tai Chi keeps you on your feet, promoting bone density.

These ancient systems are not for everyone and I suggest that many who are Yin deficient will benefit, once no longer extremely Yin deficient, from resistance and weight-training. The aim of resistance and weight-training should not at first be to build huge muscles but to build strength and resilience. The latter comes partly from cardiovascular function so some prior warm-up is vital. Take advice. (Eventually one might aim to do interval training[14] several times a week, with

14. http://www.acupuncture-points.org/interval-training.html

resistance training or weights on other days. These are subjects too big to cover here but there are links in the footnote to some sites.)

Of course, you should take advice before starting to do weight-training and you must eat more too! You may want a healthy body, but to build it you need food, and that includes carbohydrates for energy. Without enough food, you will quickly overstrain yourself and probably return to Yin deficiency.

Above all, realise that these are long-term projects, not quick fixes to be dropped when no immediate change is apparent. Of course it is possible to build strength and resilience without weights but weights are for many a better regime and done right, they build core strength too.

Failing Tai Chi, Yoga, interval training and resistance (eg weights) training, what else could you do? Possibly more convenient for many than any of the above, is the regime developed by a Royal Canadian Air-force physiotherapist in 1967. His aim was to find a simple regime that anyone in the RCAF could do, be they a pilot, a store-master or a cleaner. It had to be do-able quickly because many pilots had tight schedules. It had to be possible to do it in a small space, such as in a plane or small bedroom. It had to build resilience and cardiovascular function. Do it, and as you grow stronger, you will be able to run for buses and upstairs again without exhaustion. This is the 'XBX System for Physical Fitness' published by Penguin.

8/. Gentle, affirming massage[15] is a wonderful Yang-pacifying treatment that, particularly when practised by someone with knowledge of either Bowen technique or acupuncture points and how to use them with massage, can also enhance Yin.

---

15. http://www.acupuncture-points.org/massage.html

However, even a good (ordinary) massage from someone without such precise knowledge can be hugely beneficial.

Tuina: is a Chinese-based form of acupressure, related to Shiatsu. Since the practitioner knows acupuncture theory they can incorporate it into their treatments. Shiatsu is the Japanese equivalent.

9/ **Medication** from your doctor. This is usually given to calm excess Yang. Medication to promote Yin has not been developed as far as I am aware: this falls into the field of herbs, nutrition and nutriceuticals. Medications prescribed by doctors trained in Western medicine are usually very pure, and are either manufactured using chemicals or extracted from concentrated herbs. The aim is to isolate the so-called 'active' principal and prescribe it. This method is totally at odds with the experience of Chinese medicine which seeks to give a balanced formula.

Lacking that balance, there will nearly always be (at least) two actions by the drug. The first 'Primary' action, if the drug is considered to be successful, will be to calm the Yang. The 'Secondary' action, depending on the reaction by the body, will almost certainly be in time to deplete Yin, leading to some of the symptoms that were supposed to be treated.

Every drug has secondary effects, amongst which are symptoms similar to those for which the drug is being taken. (For more on this see my book "Qi Stagnation – Signs of Stress", chapter 8.)

10/ **Homeopathy** – low potency, often repeated until change – get advice. It is difficult when treating oneself to be objective and dispassionate when choosing the right foods or herbs. With homoeopathy it is even harder. For one thing you are searching for a homoeopathic medicine (the word always used is 'remedy') that, if given to you when healthy, would produce your current symptoms of Yin deficiency. For another, you have to choose the dosage and 'potency' to suit your particular health circumstances.

These three actions, choosing the remedy that suits the patient, then choosing the dosage and potency of the remedy, are often hard enough for a skilled homoeopath, let alone you. When you are in a weakened Yin-deficient state, whichever remedy is chosen will usually be given in low potency to be taken regularly or until some change occurs.

However, this is not a fixed rule. Sometimes a homoeopath will discern a deeper pattern in the patient's life for which a particular homoeopathic remedy is extremely relevant and suitable in a 'high' potency.

11/ **Energy healing and biofeedback**. We can now measure brainwaves to see how health, illness and stress affect them. In the 1970s I studied with one of the developers of what became known as the 'Mind Mirror'. This device measured my brainwaves by means of wires to pads at various points on my skull and showed the brainwaves produced by each side of my brain: usually they were imbalanced and I had to meditate for a long time before they began to 'mirror' one another and achieve the right shape. (On one occasion they reached it immediately. This was shortly after I'd fallen in love with someone, but unfortunately neither the romance nor the brainwave balance lasted for long!)

Among various demonstrations of how it worked was one where they attached one machine to a patient in distress and another to a healer. As the healer 'healed', both sets of brainwaves moved towards the ideal, balanced, pattern: subsequently the patient reported a huge improvement in her symptoms. This is not to suggest that you buy a 'mind mirror' machine – they are not cheap. But many forms of biofeedback can help you stabilise your brainwaves. Also, there are healers who can help you. To begin with you may need regular help but if you continue with it, at some point you will be able to maintain and build on the improvements without further help.

12/. **Breathing**. The *first* and *last* way to strengthen yin is by breathing correctly. How you breathe makes a HUGE difference to your health in general and your yin energy in particular.

In Chinese medicine, your Lungs send energy downwards – hence the reason that you are told to take a few deep breaths when you are over-emotional. So on the surface, calming your breathing sends excess energy downwards.

But your breath/energy is then said to be 'grasped' by your Kidney energy. Over time, by practising good breathing technique, you can enhance your Kidney energy and develop more Yin energy.

How do you learn to breathe properly like this? There are various ways – for example:

- Taking exercise that gets you out of breath: walking uphill is a good way!
- Hatha Yoga
- Good posture – Alexander method may show you mistakes you are making
- Buteyko breathing exercises
- Learning to meditate

I invite you to research these and choose one or more. The effort will repay itself if you apply what you learn.

Sleep

What about herbs/medications that enable people to do without sleep? Doing without sleep is not recommended. Perhaps, one day, we shall be able to take safe medications that keep us going without the need for sleep, but in general we should be aware of the Primary and Secondary effects of drugs. Although the Primary effect of such a drug is, in this case, to keep you awake indefinitely, the Secondary effect will almost certainly appear eventually. Usually the Secondary effect works in the opposite way to the Primary effect.

Finally ...

Finally any treatment that stimulates only Yin and Blood may make the condition last longer than had it also stimulated Qi and Yang. It is unwise to boost just the Yin side without also involving the Yang side. With this in mind I invite you to consider a regime that improves circulation and resilience, enhances the feel-good factor, improves alertness, brings health to your skin and improves your immune function.

It takes just a few minutes daily. It is called a cold shower, although probably cold baths are even better. There is, however, a right and a wrong way to do it.

For how to take a cold shower see http://www.acupuncture-points.org/cold-showers.html

CHAPTER 11

Conclusion

In Chinese medicine, the ultimate control of Yin and Yang is said to rest with our Kidney function[1].

This concept of Kidney does not arise in Western medicine, but it covers our long-term resources, those acquired through our genes and those we build or deplete during our lives.

Lack of these resources makes us fearful and unstable, always needing to start again.

That need to renew ourselves can be used to turn our lives around, to learn new skills and enjoy new opportunities.

So as you take time to renew your Yin resources, consider how you would like to spend the next period of your life[2].

That may become a new chapter for you.

Finally ... Your Review?

Now you've read this book, *please review it!*

As implied in the introduction, it aims to be not just informative, but *useful*.

If you think others would benefit from it, please post your opinion somewhere prospective readers might see it, such as on Amazon.

Here   are   links   to   the   North   American   site

---

1. http://www.acupuncture-points.org/kidney-function.html
2. See also Chapter 5 of 'Qi Stagnation - Signs of Stress'.

(https://www.amazon.com)   and   the   UK   site
(https://www.amazon.co.uk).

- Just click on the link above (either amazon.com or
  amazon.co.uk – or of course, your own country's equivalent)
- Put "Yuck! Phlegm!" in the search box at the top of the
  Amazon page
- When a picture of the book appears, click on where it says
  'review' or 'reviews', then
- Click on "Write a customer review" and say what you think
  about it:
- You can give it 5 stars out of 5 – if you think it merits them, of
  course!

I hope you will be positive and constructive, but if you have
major criticisms or reservations, I would like to know!

Then I can improve it for the next person.

Let me know your views, positive or otherwise, through my
website   http://www.acupuncture-points.org/yin-
deficiency.html where, towards the bottom of the page there is
a box for writing to me about your experiences and opinions.
NB *Your views will not be published without your permission.*

Thank-you!

Action Programme

Some people like action programmes and spreadsheets.

Below is a spread-sheet with suggested actions for each stage
of health improvement from severe Yin deficiency to health.

The entries are only suggestions and readers can design their
own preferred regimes.

Starting with Severe Yin Deficiency...	...What should you do and in what order?
Action	Examples

1 Calm your Mind	Take a holiday. Learn to meditate. Receive acupuncture. Take sick leave.
2. Men, reduce ejaculation. Women, fix heavy periods and get help with menopause	Men, learn the withholding method. Women – see an experienced therapist, eg an acupuncturist.
3. Get good sleep.	Get good acupuncture. Take herbs. See a doctor for medication.
4. Fix digestion and diet.	See a doctor or acupuncturist. Take time off. Study nutrition. Meet friends and eat together. Choose the right foods and learn to prepare, cook and eat them properly. Improve eating habits.
5. Get supportive therapies (but not all at once).	Acupuncture, herbs, massage, homoeopathy, Bowen technique, tuina, shiatsu ...
6. Learn to deal with stress.	Assertiveness training. Get help or advice re career or job or relationship
7. Build resilience.	Start taking cool or cold showers and begin walking and gentle exercise.
8. Exercise more vigorously.	Walk faster. Tai Qi. Yoga, Swim. Interval training. Resistance training.
9. Reassess what works.	See an acupuncturist. Talk to a friend or counsellor. Refine nutrition and eating habits.
10. Continue indefinitely, accepting that time passes ...	Watch signs of Yin deficiency recede and general health and well-being and strength improve.

Appendix 1 - Food Energetics

Before using the information in these tables read and understand Chapter 9.

NB The author and publisher accept no responsibility for results.
See an experienced practitioner for help.

A few last reminders and warnings! If, being yin deficient, you eat too many yin-enhancing foods, without sufficient yang-enhancing foods to balance them, you may find yourself getting excess yin symptoms, which include oedema, catarrh, obesity, loose stools; even cold.

This will be counter-productive. You want the food you eat to go into improving your bone tissue, enhancing your vascular and nervous systems and strengthening your immune system etc and so providing you with the security of having a body (and brain) that keeps you cool and calm and supports you firmly in life.

You may also notice, above, a few warming foods that nourish the Blood. Blood nourishing foods are usually good for Yin deficient people but even here, some Yang-type foods should be included, of which the most useful is root ginger (not dried ginger, which can be too heating.)

Individual Reactions

The above classifications are generally accepted. However, individuals have individual reactions. You may be someone for whom too many oranges, for example, seem to be heating not cooling, as described. (For example, they might produce a rash.)

In that case, your individual reaction is more important and relevant for you than what it says here. Also, there are many kinds of orange and the one that affects you may not be the same as the orange in the list (- and no, I don't know which one is listed!) So if you are not familiar with a particular food, be cautious before eating it in quantity.

Also, remember that all items listed in a given column, such as under 'cooling', are not equally cooling. To give an example, take the 'warming' column: both cumin, garlic and dates are listed as being warming, but of these garlic is probably the most warming (though it depends on the variety and bulb), cumin is next and dates are least warming.

Note: to delve into the full properties and energetics of Western herbs, I strongly recommend 'The Energetics of Western Herbs' by Peter Holmes, published by Artemis.

Food Name	Nature	Cold	Cooling	Neutral	Warming	Hot
Abalone	yang			neutral	warming	
Alfalfa	blood			neutral		
Amarinth	yin		cooling			
Angled luffa	yin	cold				
Apple	yin		cooling			
Apricot fruit	balanced			neutral		
Apricot seed	yang			neutral		
Arrowhead	yin	cold				
Artichoke	yin		cooling			
Asparagus	blood				warming	
Bamboo shoot	yin	cold				
Banana	yin	cold				
Barley	yin		cooling			
Bean(mung bean)	yin		cooling			
Bean, broad bean	balance			neutral		
Bean, sword bean	yang				warming	
Bean, kidney	balance			neutral		
Bean, string	balance			neutral		
Bean-curd, tofu	yin		cooling			

Bean, Aduki	balance			neutral	
Beef	balance			neutral	
Beetroot	balance			neutral	
Bitter gourd	yin	cold			
Black sesame seed	balance			neutral	
Broccoli	yin		cooling		
Brown sugar	yang				warming
Buckwheat	yin		cooling		
Cabbage	balance			neutral	
Cabbage (Chinese)	yin		cooling		
Cabbage (Beijing)	yin		cooling		
Caraway seed	yang				warming
Cardamon	yin				warming
Carp fish	yang			neutral	
Carrot	balance			neutral	
Cashew nut	balance			neutral	
Cauliflower	yin		cooling		
Celery	yin		cooling		
Cheese (dairy cow)	yin		cooling		
Cherry	yang				warming
Chestnut	yang				warming
Chicken	yang				warming
Chilli pepper	yang					hot
Chinese chives	yang				warming
Chives	yang				warming
Chive seed	yang				warming
Chrysanthemum	yin	cold			
Chrysanthemum, edible or 'garland'	yang				warming
Cinnamon	yang					hot

Clam	yin	cold		
Clove	yang			warming
Coconut	yin		cooling	
Coffee	yang			warming
Coix seed	yin		cooling	
Conch	yin		cooling	
Coriander	yang			warming
Corn (ie maize)	balance		neutral	
Crab	yin	cold		
Crab apple	balance		neutral	
Cream (dairy cow)	yin		cooling	
Cucumber	yin		cooling	
Cumin	yang			warming
Cuttlefish	yin		cooling	neutral
Dates	yang			warming
Dill seed	yang			warming
Duck	balance		neutral	
Duck egg	yin		cooling	
Eel (fresh water)	yang			warming
Egg white	yin		cooling	
Egg yolk	balance		neutral	
Egg plant (aubergine)	yin		cooling	
Fennel	yang			warming
Fig	balance		neutral	
Frog	yin		cooling	
Fungus ("black fungus")	balance		neutral	
Fuzzy melon	balance		neutral	
Garlic	yang			warming
Ginger (fresh root)	yang			warming

Ginger (dried powder)	yang				hot
Ginseng ("American")	balance		cooling	neutral	
Ginseng (Chinese)	yang			warming	
Goat's milk	yang			warming	
Goose	balance			neutral	
Goose egg	yang			warming	
Grapefruit	yin	cold			
Grapes	balance			neutral	
Green onion	yang			warming	
Hairtail fish	yang			warming	
Ham	yang			warming	
Honey	balance			neutral	
Horseradish	yang				hot
Iceland moss	Blood		cooling		
Irish moss	yin		cooling		
Jasmine	yang			warming	
Jellyfish (preserved)	yin	cold			
Job's tears, coix	yin		cooling		
Kelp seaweed	Blood		cooling		
Kohlrabi	balance			neutral	
Kumquat	balance			neutral	
Lamb	yang			warming	
Leaf mustard	yin		cooling		
Leeks	yang			warming	
Lemon	balance			neutral	
Lettuce	yin	cold			
Lettuce (Indian)	yin		cooling		
Lettuce root	yin		cooling		
Licorice root (raw)	balance			neutral	warming

Lily bulb	yin		cooling	
Lily flower	yin		cooling	
Liver of pig	yang			warming
Loach	balance		neutral	
Lobster	yang			warming
Longan fruit	yang			warming
Loquat fruit	yin		cooling	
Lotus root	yin	cold		
Lotus seed	balance		neutral	
Luffa fruit, loofah	yin		cooling	
Lychee fruit	yang			warming
Maltose	yang			warming
Mandarin orange	yin		cooling	
Mango	yin		cooling	
Marjoram	yin		cooling	
Micro-algae	Blood		neutral	
Milk (cow's milk)	balance		neutral	
Millet	yin		cooling	
Mulberry	yin	cold		
Mushroom	yin		cooling	
Mushroom, tremelia	balance		cooling	
Musk melon	yin		cooling	
Mussels	yang			warming
Mustard seed	yang				hot
Mutton	yang			warming
Nettle	Blood		cooling	
Nutmeg	yang			warming
Oats	Blood			warming
Olives	balance		neutral	

Onion	yang				warming	
Orange	yin		cooling			
Osmanthus flowers	yang				warming	
Oyster	balance			neutral		
Papaya	yin		cooling			
Pea	yin		cooling			
Peach	yang				warming	
Peanut (unroasted)	balance			neutral		
Peanut, roasted	yang					hot
Pears	yin		cooling			
Pepper, black	yang					hot
Peppercorn, 'Sichuan'	yang				warming	
Peppermint	yang				warming	
Persimmon	yin	cold				
Pig skin	yin		cooling			
Pig's bone marrow	yin	cold				
Pine nut	yang				warming	
Pineapple	yin		cooling			
Pistachio nut	balance			neutral		
Plums	balance			neutral		
Pollen (from flowers)	Blood		cooling	neutral		
Pomengranate	yang				warming	
Pomelo (lusho fruit)	yin	cold				
Pork meat	balance			neutral	warming	
Potato	balance			neutral		
Pumpkin	balance			neutral		
Quail flesh	balance			neutral		
Quail egg	balance			neutral		
Rabbit meat	yin		cooling			

Radish (Chinese)	yin		cooling		
Radish leaf	balance			neutral	
Raspberry	yang				warming
Rhubarb	yin	cold			
Rice, glutinous	yang				warming
Rice, round-grained	balance			neutral	
Rock sugar	balance			neutral	
Root of kudzu vine	yin	cold			
Rose bud	yang				warming
Rosemary	yang				warming
Royal jelly honey	balance			neutral	
Sage	yin		cooling		
Salt	yin	cold			
Sea clams	yin	cold			
Sea cucumber	yang				warming
Sea eels	balance			neutral	
Sea shrimp	balance			neutral	
Seaweed	yin	cold	cooling		
Sesame oil	yin		cooling		
Shiitake mushroom	balance			neutral	
Shrimps, fresh water	yang				warming
Snails	yin	cold			
Soya sauce	yin	cold			
Soybean milk	balance			neutral	
Soybean oil	yang					hot
Soybeans	balance			neutral	
Sparrow	yang				warming
Sparrow egg	yang				warming
Spearmint	yang				warming

Spinach	yin		cooling	
Sprouts	yin	cold		
Squash	yang			warming
Star anise	yang			warming
Star fruit (carambola)	yin	cold		
Strawberry	yin		cooling	
Sugar molasses	yang			warming
Sugar cane	yin	cold		
Sunflower seed	balance		neutral	warming
Sweet basil	yang			warming
Sweet pepper	yang			warming
Sweet potato	balance		neutral	
Sword bean	yang			warming
Tangerine	yin		cooling	
Taro	balance		neutral	
Tea (Indian or Chinese)	yin		cooling	
Thyme	yang			warming
Tobacco	yang			warming
Tofu, bean-curd	yin		cooling	
Tomato	yin	cold		
Turnips	balance		neutral	
Vegetable oil	yang			warming
Vegetables, green	Blood			warming
Venison	yang			warming
Vinegar	yang			warming
Walnut	yang			warming
Water caltrop	yin		cooling	
Water chestnut	yin	cold		
Water spinach	yin	cold		

Watercress	Blood	cold		neutral
Watermelon	yin	cold		
Wax gourd	yin		cooling	
Wheat	yin		cooling	
Wheat-grass	Blood			neutral
Wild rice stem	yin	cold		
Wild yam	Blood			neutral
Wine	yang			warming
yogurt (dairy cow)	yin		cooling	

Appendix 2 - Recipes for Yin Deficiency

Inventive cooks will have no difficulty thinking of recipes that benefit people with Yin deficiency. By and large they will be recipes that favour:

- Green vegetables (for Blood), not overcooked
- Protein (for Blood) to build muscle, not fat
- Root vegetables (for Yin), not overcooked
- Natural oils, both saturated and unsaturated, the former because our genes are used to them and the latter because we cannot manufacture all the oils we need without them

They will NOT include many foods that are quickly turned into sugars when digested such as:

- Refined grain-based foods, for example white bread, white flour, biscuits, cakes
- Other foods, some of them root vegetables, that easily transform into sugars (potato, for example)
- Sugar: be careful not to eat too much fruit, rich in sugars
- Alcoholic and other drinks, eg fruit juices, heavy in sugars and flavourings or stimulants
  NOR will they include foods that over-stimulate:

- Caffeine and other stimulants that draw on Yin reserves to create the 'buzz' and sense of invincibility or power or joy
- Highly spiced foods that dissipate Qi

So, what remains may seem relatively boring! For people who have become dependent on sugars and caffeine-type foods that maintain a constant 'wired alertness' these recipes may initially seem to lower your energy.

But, given time and perseverance you will find that you sleep better, your recover from stressful situations more quickly, you are more relaxed yet just as alert as before, but less nervous about your performance. In effect, you will become more resilient and confident.

On the following pages are examples of recipes that can be said to benefit people with Yin deficiency. Some of them include foods that taken in quantity on their own would emphasise Yang too much, but taken as part of the recipe they balance the Yin side of it.

Although it is possible to be vegetarian and eat a Yin enhancing meal, it is faster to include protein from animal sources. (However, ideally they should be free from antibiotics and steroids, and have been bred on organic foodstuffs. So in effect they should be what in the UK is classified as *organic*.)

Foods such as vegetables should not be over-cooked.

Do not eat always the same food or recipe. Every food has its own qualities and nutrients and for health you need a wide range of resources.

To start with avoid raw, uncooked and chilled or frozen foods because these strain your Yang resources to digest.

Cooking provides a Yang element to what you eat; some methods of cooking such as roasting and stir-frying, in particular. Any way of cooking that increases the water-content of the food may increase its Yin quality but possibly make it harder for Yang to metabolise.

Do not forget that food is only one way of improving your health. Sleep, exercise and other methods explained in this book all contribute. On its own, the right diet will improve your health only slowly.

As you grow fitter, ie more balanced as between Yin and Yang, you can afford to eat a wider range of foods, and when you return to health you may even eat some junk foods occasionally!

If you are very cold, or the weather is very cold, you should include more Yang foods than normal because your aim is always to support your body's ability to absorb what you eat. Equally, on very hot days, you may be able to eat foods with less Yang in them.

Chewing

Whatever you eat, get into the habit of chewing it well before you swallow it. Chewing is a Yang process that supports your Stomach and Spleen when they come to digesting your food and transforming it into Blood and Yin.

Chewing also slows you down! Chewing is an exercise that helps your dissipate stress. Chew well!

Fish Dishes

Fish containing natural unsaturated oils is a great food for Yin deficiency people. Unfortunately, many fish are farmed so have been subjected to heavy doses of fungicides and pesticides. Many oceans are being over-fished and some seas are high in impurities and heavy metals, so even line-caught 'natural' ocean fish may not be perfect.

Simple preparation in foil
Almost any fish can be quickly prepared by gutting it, removing its head and tail, and wrapping in foil with a few additions such as lemon juice and salt. If the fish is fresh, a few minutes in the oven will produce a wonderful and nutritious food. Add cooked green vegetables.

Fish and chips
Even fish and chips is not all bad. Admittedly the chips are heavier in saturated fats than desirable, but at least those fats retard how fast the carbohydrate is absorbed, and the fish is served with vegetables, which should be eaten rather than pushed aside. However, the saturated fats here can be fairly heating so fish and chips should be eaten only occasionally.

Crab meat wrapped in Sole (enough for 4 people)

- 4 fillets of sole
- 200gms (approx ½ pound) cooked crab meat, chopped finely
- 2 tablespoons finely chopped onions
- 4 tablespoons butter, melted
- 1 cup chicken broth
- 2 tablespoons fresh lemon juice
- 1 cup dry white wine
- 1 tablespoon arrowroot for thickening
- Lemon wedges and parsley for garnish
- Salt and pepper

- A shallow baking pan

- Wooden toothpicks

Turn on the oven, to heat to 375F or 190C.

Divide the crab-meat into four roughly equal amounts. Roll each up in one of the sole fillets, securing the rolled fish with one or more toothpicks. Pour the melted butter into the baking pain and place the rolled fillets side by side in it. Sprinkle on the onion.

Combine the wine, broth and lemon juice and pour around and over the fillets. Add salt and a little ground pepper. Place in the oven and bake for 12 minutes.

Transfer the fillets to a serving platter and pour the remaining fluid into a saucepan or, if the baking platter can be heated on the hob, simmer the fluid until it reduces to 2/3 cup. Dissolve arrowroot in 2 tablespoons of this fluid and stir into the remaining sauce. Cook, stirring, until it thickens and pour the fluid over the fish. Serve with garnish and a cooked green vegetable such as broccoli.

Salmon in Poacher's Pouch with Rice and Peas

- 4 x 175gm (6 oz) Salmon steaks or cutlets

- 2 medium carrots, cut into Julienne strips (ie,very thin)

- 1 yellow pepper, de-seeded, cut into thin strips

- 1 medium leek, shredded

- 2 medium oranges

- 2 spring onions (or shallots) finely sliced

- 3 tablespoons of soya sauce

- Sprig of Parsley as garnish (optional)

- 4 pieces of either grease-proof or baking paper, each 18" sq (Do not use cling-film.)

Mix the carrot, pepper and leek strips together. Divide into 4 piles, one each in the centre of a grease-proof or baking paper. Place a salmon cutlet or steak on each of the vegetable piles.

Into a glass, squeeze the juice of the oranges and then add the pulp of the orange (not the rind). Add the soya sauce and mix. Spoon the mixture over the salmon cutlets/steaks. Scatter on the sliced onions.

Bring the sides of the paper together, fold together and then taper the ends and fold under the salmon and vegetables, making a neat parcel of each.

Place in the steamer and steam for 9 minutes or microwave for 4 ½ minutes. Serve with brown rice and peas, sprinkling on the garnish.

Note: the brown rice takes longer to cook and only half a cup of the cooked rice should be served with each salmon parcel. A good way to cook the brown rice, making it more digestible, is to gently fry a sliced onion in a saucepan in olive or coconut oil, then add the washed rice with a sprinkling of ground, dried seaweed. Meanwhile boil up enough water or chicken stock to cover the rice with an extra half inch on top.

Pour the boiling water/stock into the rice, stir and cover to simmer for 30 minutes by when the rice should have been absorbed all the stock.

Baked Herring fillets with Fennel and Coriander

- 455gms (1lb) herring fillets

- 1 small fennel bulb, thinly sliced

- ½ small red onion, sliced

- Salt and pepper

- 1 x 15ml spoon (1 tablespoon) balsamic vinegar

- 1 x 15ml (1 tablespoon) fresh chopped coriander

- Pinch of brown sugar

1. Lay each fillet onto a large square of baking parchment or foil.
2. Add the fennel, onion, oil, seasoning, vinegar, coriander and sugar.
3. Fold the baking parchment or foil to make a parcel and place onto a baking tray.
4. Cook for 15-20 minutes (180C) and serve with salad.

Cullen Skink (serves 4)

This is a traditional Scottish soup made with smoked fish. Smoking slightly increases the Yang quality of the dish but otherwise it is broadly speaking neutral, so fine for tonifying Yin. However, it may not suit people who are milk intolerant, although the presence of the onion often makes the milk acceptable to them.

- 455gms (1 lb) smoked fish, chopped into smallish chunks
- 2 medium onions, sliced
- 1 pint of milk
- 1 tablespoon of coconut or olive oil
- Salt and pepper, and herbs – but the dish is fine without them
- Optional – 2 medium potatoes, lightly boiled and chopped into quarters (keep the skins on them ie do not discard the skins)

Gently brown the onions in the oil. Add the milk and bring to the boil. Add the fish, potato. Salt and pepper and herbs, if any. Simmer for at least 15 minutes.

For more ideas, see our website
http://www.acupuncture-points.org/yin-deficiency-recipes.html

Appendix 3 - Complications

When you may need professional help

1. **Damp** is a Yin excess[1] problem. (For more about Damp see http://www.acupuncture-points.org/damp.html.) You can have Damp at the same time as being Yin deficient, meaning it is possible to have both excess Yin and deficient Yin at the same time.

Unfortunately, many treatments for Yin deficiency will make your Damp worse so your options diet-wise are more restricted as many Yin enhancing foods are also moisturising, which worsens Damp. This is where professional help may be necessary to sort out the best way forward.

2. **Phlegm**[2] is a stronger form of Yin even than Damp. It is certainly possible to have Phlegm as well as Yin deficiency which, if there is also Deficiency Heat, engenders more Phlegm, a vicious cycle. Here the Phlegm must be cleared before returning to deal with the Yin deficiency, because efforts to clear the Yin deficiency may easily worsen the Phlegm.

Phlegm is insidious and can be hard to clear. The fourth book in this series on *Chinese Medicine in English* is on Phlegm and how to understand and deal with it.

3. **Infections** can cause a sensation of Heat[3] such as with a fever, but for some people they experience this as Cold, even though the thermometer says they have a fever. If the sensation is predominantly of Heat, then the attack will probably be short and may even stimulate your body to deal with its Yin deficiency. However, if the attack and sensation of Heat lasts a long time then it can seriously exhaust or 'consume' your Yin resources. The right treatment may need careful consideration. If the predominant sensation during the fever is of Cold, then probably you are deficient in both Yin and Yang: further complications!

See http://www.acupuncture-points.org/external-heat and-cold.html.

Should you be interested in how Chinese medicine explains and treats

1. See http://www.acupuncture-points.org/yin-excess.html
2. http://www.acupuncture-points.org/phlegm.html
3. See also http://www.acupuncture-points.org/Heat.html

diseases of an exterior origin, such as come from bacteria and viruses, be prepared for quite a read. It has been the subject of considerable thought over perhaps 15 centuries! On my website I summarise this on two pages:

- http://www.acupuncture-points.org/four-levels.html

- http://www.acupuncture-points.org/six-stages.html

4. **Cold**[4] 'invasion'. As in 2/ above, if you experience an 'attack' of Cold, a Yin 'evil', the appropriate treatment in Chinese medicine is to clear the Cold before returning to treat the Yin deficiency.

5. **Heat**. Heat in the environment can deplete your Yin energy. Avoid hot climates or conditions such as saunas and steam rooms, very warm central-heating and foods that are too warming. (On the other hand, ice-cold air- conditioning won't help much either, because it may make you so cold your body can't engender the heat necessary to mend itself.)

6. **Lack of Yang** . As in 4/ above, you do need some Yang to mend your Yin. Too much Yang is counterproductive, but so is too little! If you are deficient in both Yin and Yang (as you may be, lacking only slightly less Yang than Yin), this is where careful treatment may include some element of Yang. Better to get help than try to do it yourself.

7. **Internal Heat**. This is sometimes a real problem, which I've often seen. It is worse when the patient is old, because he or she lacks enough energy and time to get better.

It often follows an infection or debilitating condition such as shingles or HIV. The internal Heat is like a labouring car engine in a heatwave when the passengers insist on having the air-conditioning on but this uses up all the car's power, and the fuel tank is emptying fast.

Any improvement in Yin – the fuel supply – is immediately used up fighting the Heat. Treatment requires measures to quell the empty Heat and to build Yin. This can be difficult and, in old people, there may be little time. However, in younger people, the fact that there is a clear treatment programme usually leads to success.

4. See http://www.acupuncture-points.org/cold.html

Appendix 4 – References

DVD 'Sweet Misery – A Poisoned World' https://topdocumentaryfilms.com/sweet-misery-a-poisoned-world/

Books

- The End of Time – Julian Barbour, Phoenix 1999
- The Energetics of Western Herbs – Peter Holmes, Artemis 1989
- Qi Stagnation – Signs of Stress – Jonathan Clogstoun-Willmott, Frame of Mind Publishing 2013
- Yang Deficiency – Get Your Fire Burning Again! – Jonathan Clogstoun-Willmott, Frame of Mind Publishing 2016
- Physical Fitness: 5BX 11-minute-a-day plan for men, XBX 12-minute-a-day plan for women by by Royal Canadian Air Force (Penguin)
- The Golden Needle – Richard Bertschinger, Churchill Livingstone 1991
- Foundations of Chinese Medicine – Giovanni Maciocia, Churchill Livingstone, 2005
- Chinese System of Food Cures – H Liu, Sterling 1968
- The Search for Modern China, Jonathan Spence, Norton 1999

- Authentic I Ching, Henry Wei, Softback Preview 1993
- I Ching, Book of Change, John Blofeld, Unwin 1980
- Yin-Yang Code, Ning Lu PhD, Universe Books 2008
- Tao of Health, Sex & Longevity, Daniel Reid, Fireside 1989

Articles, letters

- 'Cooking and Transfats' on letters page of Scientific American July 2014.

Links

- http://www.acupuncture-points.org
- http://www.mercola.com

Appendix 5 - Books by Jonathan Clogstoun-Willmott

Chinese Medicine in English Series published by *Frame of Mind Publishing*

- Qi Stagnation – Signs of Stress, 2013
- Yin Deficiency – Burnout and Exhaustion – What to Do! 2014
- Yang Deficiency – Get your Fire Burning Again! 2016
- Yuck! Phlegm! How to Clear your Phlegm using ideas from Chinese Medicine 2017

Originally published by Aquarius

- Western Astrology and Chinese Medicine, 1986

Appendix 6 – the author

Jonathan Clogstoun-Willmott has been practising Chinese medicine and acupuncture since 1979. He has taught Chinese medicine since 1985 and his website http://www.acupuncture-points.org explaining Chinese medicine in layman's English attracts praise from round the world.